D1605591

420

MEDITATIONS

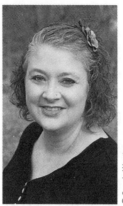
© Connie Wurster

About the Author

Kerri Connor has been practicing her craft for over thirty-five years and has run an eclectic Pagan family group, the Gathering Grove, since 2003.

She is a frequent contributor to Llewellyn annuals and is the author of *Wake, Bake & Meditate: Take Your Spiritual Practice to a Higher Level with Cannabis*. Kerri runs the Spiral Labyrinth, a mini spiritual retreat, at her home in Ringwood, IL.

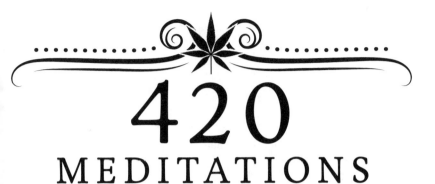

420

MEDITATIONS

Enhance Your Spiritual Practice
❖ With Cannabis ❖

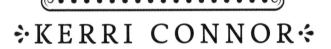

❖ KERRI CONNOR ❖

Llewellyn Publications
Woodbury, Minnesota

FIRST EDITION
Third Printing, 2021

Book design by Samantha Peterson
Cover design by Shira Atakpu
Llewellyn Publications is a registered trademark of Llewellyn Worldwide Ltd.

Library of Congress Cataloging-in-Publication Data
Names: Connor, Kerri, author.
Title: 420 meditations : enhance your spiritual practice with cannabis /
   Kerri Connor.
Other titles: Four hundred and twenty meditations
Description: First edition. | Woodbury, Minnesota : Llewellyn Worldwide, Ltd, 2021. |
   Includes bibliographical references. | Summary: "The meditations in this book have
   been designed to enhance the reader's spiritual journey and integrate the profound
   feelings, healing energies, and wise insights of cannabis."—Provided by publisher.
Identifiers: LCCN 2020051533 (print) | LCCN 2020051534 (ebook) |
   ISBN 9780738765280 | ISBN 9780738765471 (ebook)
Subjects: LCSH: Hallucinogenic drugs and religious experience. | Cannabis.| Meditations.
Classification: LCC BL65.D7 C66 2021 (print) | LCC BL65.D7 (ebook) | DDC
   204/.35—dc23
LC record available at https://lccn.loc.gov/2020051533
LC ebook record available at https://lccn.loc.gov/2020051534

Llewellyn Publications
A Division of Llewellyn Worldwide Ltd.
2143 Wooddale Drive
Woodbury, MN 55125-2989
www.llewellyn.com

Other Books by Kerri Connor

Ostara (Llewellyn Publications)

Spells for Tough Times (Llewellyn Publications)

*The Pocket Spell Creator: Magickal References
at Your Fingertips* (New Page Books)

*The Pocket Guide to Rituals: Magickal References
at Your Fingertips* (New Page Books)

The Pocket Idiot's Guide to Potions (Alpha Books)

*Wake, Bake & Meditate: Take Your Spiritual Practice to a
Higher Level with Cannabis* (Llewellyn Publications)

For the Gathering Grove

Contents

Disclaimer

Using, distributing, or selling cannabis is a federal crime, and may also be illegal in your state or local vicinity. It is your responsibility to understand all laws pertaining to the possession or use of cannabis. Neither the author nor publisher are accountable for consequences derived from the possession or use thereof.

Always seek the advice of a qualified health provider regarding medical questions.

This book is not a substitute for medical advice.

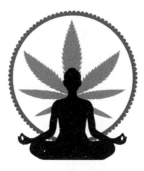

Introduction

While writing *Wake, Bake & Meditate: Take Your Spiritual Practice to a Higher Level with Cannabis*, I knew I had to do this second book to show how easily you can incorporate weed-inspired meditation into your daily life with a more relaxed, less ritualistic approach that still combines cannabis, meditation, and a bit of magic all into one. In this book, you do not need to seek a peak experience for each meditation. You may perform them lightly buzzed or in a much deeper state, but a peak experience is not the overall goal for most of these. There will be a few meditations where it is noted a peak experience is ideal.

What is a peak experience? If you have not heard of a peak experience before, the best way to describe it is this: A peak experience with the use of cannabis is when you reach a level in your high where you feel completely at one with the universe. You feel there are no boundaries separating you from the environment around you. It is the ultimate feeling of oneness and makes for an ideal setting for connection and communion with the divine, universe, spiritual guides, or your higher self.

Cannabis can complement your work in many ways, and while the first book centered on the more ritualistic approach, which I believe greatly helps beginners as they are getting started, this book brings weed-assisted meditation into your daily life to be used at any time. Cannabis allows users to get in touch with themselves. It assists the user in stepping outside of themselves to take a more objective look at themselves and their situations. It reveals thoughts and feelings, and sometimes gives you a punch to the gut with what you learn about yourself. It is an eye opener. It wakes you up.

For the most part, these meditations are not written in a guided format. Many give you questions to contemplate in your meditation. If you are meditating daily on your own, guided is a hassle. Read through the meditation, several times if necessary, and then center your focus on what you just read. Go to the place you need to go, reflect on what you need to reflect on, visualize what you need to visualize.

This book will be broken down into different sections that, overall, will cover meditations for:

- 366 days of the year
- 27 lunar meditations
- 6 solar meditations
- 8 sabbats
- 5 elemental meditations
- 8 aura and chakra meditations

The first section is set up in calendar format: January through December with each date listed. These meditations follow the cycle of the year, with each month incorporating quotes, herbs, gemstones, sounds from nature, breathwork, trance dance, meditative songs, a tasting experience, aromatherapy, and chants, along with more traditional meditations. Cannabis amplifies your senses. These meditations will help to incorporate all your senses into your spiritual practice. You don't often use other senses in a meditation, so incorporating things such as touch, scent, and taste builds on to the experience.

The special meditations you will find each month include:

- Smoke the herb: creating a mix by combining cannabis with a specific herb.

- Inspirational inklings: quotes to reflect on.
- Get stoned: working with gemstones and crystals.
- Call of the wild: connecting with sounds from nature.
- Got the munchies: working with the sense of taste.
- Chants: traditional and original chants to focus energies.
- Trance dance: having fun, moving the body, and finding a groove.
- Chill lounge: meditative songs to relate with.
- Breathe it in: working with essential oils to elicit aromatherapy benefits.
- Breathwork: grounding breathwork done to wrap up the month.

At the beginning of each month, you will find a shopping list for items you will need to correspond with some of the meditations. Stones and gems do not have to be expensive ones! Rough or tumbled stones are fine and do not have to be cut jewelry pieces; however, if you happen to have a certain stone in a piece of jewelry, you can use that in the meditation. Herbs you need can be bought in small one-ounce packages. The first week of each month will be "additional supplies" free, giving you at least a week to pick up anything you need. Crystals and herbs may be purchased at metaphysical stores, but you must ensure your herbs are "food grade." This may require some effort on your part. Many food grade herbs can be found right in your local supermarket in the spice isle. Others, like lavender and rose petals may be more difficult to find in food grade. If you have a culinary market near you, you can find these there, or you will need to order off the internet. Be sure to include the words "food grade" in your internet search. Food grade herbs are far safer for consumption. Organic food grade is even better. Always feel free to look ahead at future months for shopping lists.

Each month, you will have a meditation to do with food: "Got the munchies." Feel free to substitute similar food types if you want due to allergies or personal preferences.

When working with essential oil, if you plan on applying it to your skin at all, be sure to always use a carrier oil such as jojoba, grapeseed, or almond. There are dozens of carriers you can choose from. It is not safe to use straight essential oils on your skin, as they may cause irritations or even burns. If you are doing more than sniffing from an open bottle, be sure to protect yourself. Two to three drops of essential oil to four ounces of carrier oil works well.

Music will not be included in these shopping lists, as you will just have to perform a simple search to find the songs and suggested sounds. Be sure to check the time on your songs; if you want a longer meditation, set the song to repeat.

Some of the daily meditations are based on quotes; some may be inspirational, others are from famous pot smokers. All are designed to build your spiritual and magical relationship with cannabis.

You can pick up this book at any time and perform the meditation for the specific date. If you buy this book in September, then you start with September. You can practice every day, or you can skip days. This is your practice and therefore entirely up to you. Unless otherwise stated, all meditations begin with you getting stoned first. A few meditations will begin with directions to follow before getting stoned, but if no other instructions are stated, then light up first. This book is based on the seasons in the northern hemisphere, so our southern friends will need to simply reverse the seasonal meditations.

The subsequent sections contain meditations based on astronomical and other natural occurrences and their correspondences. This is where you will find the meditations for moons, sabbats, eclipses, solstices, chakras, elemental workings, and your birthday. By their own design, these meditations will be more spiritual in nature.

I highly suggest enhancing your meditations with music and scents of your choice when another one isn't specifically called for. Music and incense or oils help to create the perfect groove with oneness.

I can't stress enough the importance of journaling after a meditation is complete. Cannabis is wonderful. It can also play with your memory. Be sure to jot down thoughts, revelations, or other important messages you receive. You might not remember them later.

I want to thank you for joining me on this journey. Some days we will laugh together, some days we may cry, but always know you are never alone or on your own. Your guides, your protector spirits, angels, guardians, however you see them, are always there, as are your fellow supporters. You can join the Facebook group "Wake, Bake, and Meditate" for more support in your journey. You can follow me on Facebook: "@AuthorKerriConnor," or "@TheWeedWitchAuthor." My official website can be found at www.kerriconnor.com.

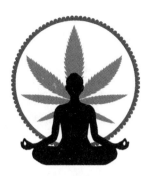

Chapter 1
366 Daily Meditations

✹ JANUARY SHOPPING LIST ✹

Garnet (January 9)

Your favorite candy/sweet treat (January 11)

Dried thyme (January 24)

Eucalyptus essential oil (January 28)

January 1
Happy New Year

New Year's Day is often a day of making resolutions, generally followed by weeks of suffering for whatever reason as you fight against what you are used to, only to fall back into old habits. Instead of making resolutions, set goals to work on.

Setting goals is different from resolutions, as it offers more self-support. How? Think of it this way: If I set a resolution to stop smoking and I mess up, my resolution is blown. But if I set a goal to not smoke for two weeks and I mess up, I try again. People simply associate resolutions not only with New Year's but with failure. Goals you can set or change at any time. Sometimes we need to be easier on ourselves to be successful.

Renew.

Reinvent.

Re-create.

These are all alternatives to resolutions.

Meditate on how incorporating these words and setting goals can help you achieve your full potential.

January 2

Inspirational inklings

"In a society that profits from your self doubt, liking your self is a rebellious act."

—Caroline Caldwell, artist and author[1]

---

1. Twitter, May 17, 2015, https://twitter.com/dirt_worship/status/6000 28189113581569?lang=en.

The world wants to always tell us what is wrong with us. Products are sold by appealing to our fears and self-doubt. Manufacturers tell us through advertising how their product can help us overcome the very self-doubt they work so hard to create. We don't have to let them. We have the choice to look in the mirror and like what we see, not only physically but emotionally, mentally, and spiritually. What do you like about yourself? What are your best qualities? Do not focus on any negatives. This mediation is only for the positives.

January 3
Your home is your castle
We have all heard the saying "your home is your castle," so today let's explore what your castle would look like. Exercise your imagination; not only is money no object, there are no limits whatsoever. Your castle can be in the clouds, on another planet, or under the sea. Where will you put your castle? What does it look like? How is it decorated? What do you do inside of it? Let yourself go and experience your one-of-a-kind home.

January 4
Self-portrait
For this meditation you will need a mirror, either hand-held or something you can comfortably sit in front of.

Look into the mirror at yourself.

Stare deeply into your own eyes. Look at your skin. Your eyebrows. Your nose. Your lips.

What do you see? Which is your favorite facial feature?

You are unique. You are the perfect you.

Examine yourself and paint your own self portrait in your meditation.

January 5
Understanding

Check out any social media app these days, and you can easily tell "understanding" has quickly become a remnant of the past. We don't listen to each other anymore. We argue, we fight, we demand.

We don't comprehend.

We see what we want to see and then decide what the other person is trying to say.

But we don't understand.

How can you improve your skills of understanding others?

How can you improve your approach so others can understand you better?

How would your life change if there was more understanding in your world?

January 6
Have faith in the world
Some days, we turn on the news and just want to cry. Here's an idea. Don't turn on the news today. Have faith in the world. Meditate on what this looks like for you. What does a world that does the "right" thing look like to you? Spend some time in this world and re-create it in your meditations whenever you feel the world is out of control. Find your peace in it where you can. Feel free to use this meditation any day when the news gets to be just too much to deal with. Take a break and walk away to recharge.

January 7
Do not seek the light; realize you are the light
We often want others to fix things for us. We see problems in the world and wonder why someone doesn't change them. It's time to take the responsibility for ourselves. What can you do to be the light in your own world? In someone else's world? What can you do to make things better? What one idea can you implement or change to make life better? Meditate on what darkness you see and how can you be the light to chase it away.

January 8
Find comfort inside

The dark half of the year is the perfect time to work on your inner self. This can include many aspects. Use today's meditation to look inside yourself. What about yourself brings you comfort? Do not focus on any negative qualities. For today, only focus on the positive. How can you soothe yourself and your soul on your own, with no help from others or from the outside world? Find this comfort inside of you and pull it out into the mundane world when you need it.

January 9
Get stoned: garnet

Garnet is a beautiful red stone that resonates with strength, protection, healing, physical energy, compassion, and purification.

Pick one of these qualities that calls to you. What do you need to call into your life? Get into your comfy spot and hold the stone in your hand out in front of you.

Examine the stone with your eyes and your fingers.

Feel the stone as you hold it tightly in your hand.

Hold the stone close to your heart.

Meditate on the stone and how it feels to you.

Feel a connection with the stone. Charge your stone by imagining it filled with that quality you seek.

Do you need strength for an upcoming project at work? Has your energy supply been lagging lately, and you could use a little boost to your physical energy? Have you been known to show a lack of compassion? Are you willing to change?

Feel the attribute you want to work with present in your stone.

Carry this stone with you whenever you feel the need.

January 10
Call of the wild: wolf song
Do an online search for "wolves howling."

Find a clip that is a good length for your meditation time or use a repeat feature.

Play the song and meditate on it as you listen.

Do you like this sound? Dislike the sound?

Let the sound encompass you.

How does it make you feel?

January 11
Got the munchies: sweet tooth
Life is often about the little things. The things we take for granted and need to learn to appreciate more. Today, get stoned, grab your candy or sweet treat, and enjoy it. But as you enjoy it, think about how it makes you feel. Does this treat have special meaning or memories for you? Is it

a new favorite? Really take the time to savor and appreciate the treat you picked out, but also connect with why you enjoy it.

January 12
Mindful breathing
Breathing is literally what keeps us alive, yet we take this essential bodily function for granted.

While breathing as you normally do, pay attention to your breath for several minutes. Don't alter it, only observe. Lay one hand on your chest and the other on your stomach to feel the movement as you inhale and exhale,

Begin increasing the depth and length of your breath.

Inhale deeply through your nose for a count of five, hold for five, then exhale through your mouth for five. Allow your breath to come out in a "whoosh." Repeat your five-count breath throughout this exercise.

Feel your stomach and chest rise and fall with each inhalation and exhalation.

Envision good air in, bad air out.

Whenever you need a pick me up, or a moment to chill, use this meditation to calm yourself, reset your breathwork, and put yourself into a better mindset.

January 13
The sound of silence

We are bombarded daily with so many sounds, absolute silence is almost an impossibility, making it seldom experienced. Spend some time in the silence you have created. Let it wash over you, cleansing away negativities. Enjoy the peace of the sound of silence while you can.

For this meditation you may need to change your normal location if there is frequent background noise.

While you might not be able to eliminate all background sounds, do the best you can. If you have earplugs, they may help you create an atmosphere of silence.

Identify and acknowledge the sounds you do hear, and then put them aside, back into the background. Focus on silence. How does it make you feel?

Some people love silence while others find it uncomfortable and off-putting. Find a place in the silence where you are comfortable.

January 14
Learning to be loved

Sadly, there are many people in the world who have a difficult time accepting love from others, because they never learned how. They were not given love to ever know how to accept it.

True love comes without strings attached; it is unconditional. Human beings are not used to that. We often feel being loved comes with expectations. When we don't know what those expectations are, we have a difficult time accepting love and instead, second-guess it and wonder when the other shoe will drop.

We may second-guess ourselves, wondering what the motives of the other person are: what is it they see that we don't?

We may feel anxious and try to figure out what is expected of us.

We may feel unworthy.

Meditate on how you accept love. Are you able to or do you have walls protecting you? Is it easy or difficult for you?

Are you open to being loved or do you block it to protect yourself from possible future heartache?

Allowing yourself to be loved requires you to be open and accepting of both yourself and others.

Do you have areas you need to work on?

January 15
Work where it hurts
The easiest way to learn what you need to work on in your life is to go directly to what hurts the most.

What has caused you the most pain in your life? Is it an ongoing situation or is it in the past but still rearing its ugly head?

Where pain resides, unhappiness does too.

While it is not possible to physically remove some situations from your life, if it is possible, then you need to work on removing it.

Meditate on where you hurt the most. What do you need to do to remove the hurt and pain? What actions can you take to protect yourself from this pain? What do you need in order to move on and put the past in the past?

January 16
Fear has a function

Fear is our mind's way of protecting us from harm by making us feel uncomfortable to do something. Often, it's from physical harm, but it can protect us from emotional harm as well. What fears do you possess that protect you emotionally? How do those fears surface in your relationships? Are they keeping you safe? Are they preventing you from moving forward or growing? Evaluate your fears. Are there ones you can now deal with and pack away? Are there ones you want to work on facing? If not, it's fine. Simply use this meditation to evaluate your fears, and acknowledge they are there.

January 17
Inspirational inklings

"What is really hard, and really amazing, is giving up on being perfect and beginning the work of becoming yourself."

—Anna Quindlen[2]

We do not need to work toward being anyone's ideal of perfection. We are all unique and perfect just as we are. Instead of working toward some generic definition of perfection, what can you do to set those standards aside and celebrate the realness, the uniqueness, the perfection of you?

January 18
Chill lounge

We are a month into winter. The nights are short, the days are gray. Wishing for warmer days and sunshine begins to settle in more deeply. We begin looking for a glimpse of the light at the end of the tunnel. What song expresses this feeling for you? What song gives you a glimpse of better days to come while still acknowledging the darkness of the present?

I use "Aurora Borealis" by Brandon Fiechter for this exercise.

---

2. Anna Quindlen, *Being Perfect* (New York: Random House), 9.

Play your music while you are in your comfy spot. Let not only the music but any lyrics flow over you, and listen deeply and intently. Where does the music take you? How does it make you feel?

January 19
Chant
"The light I see is the light I will be."

Yesterday's meditation worked with seeing the light at the end of the tunnel. Today, become one with the light and the end of the tunnel. Know that at any time, you can be the light to pull yourself through the dark.

Repeat this chant throughout your meditation.

Try saying it in different intonations and at different speeds until you find your match.

How does this chant make you feel?

January 20
Tools for change
Change is seldom easy. We cling to what we know and fear what we don't. Even when we know the change is for the better, apprehension and anxiety can set in. People may feel change is a personal criticism or rebuke, but that is not always the case.

How do you deal with change? Do you find you accept it easily, or do you struggle with it?

What tools do you have to help you deal with change? (For example, patience.) What tools do you need to develop to help you deal with change?

January 21

Snow day

You have been doing a lot of inner work. Today, no matter where you live, you get a snow day!

Today, meditate on playing and having fun in snow.

If you haven't ever done that before, find some videos and watch them first! What would you like to do in the snow? Ski? Snowboard? Make a snowman? Have a snowball fight? How do you think it would feel? Taste? Smell?

If you haven't really played in the snow for a long time, think about how it made you feel when you did. What did you like to do?

If you happen to have snow available, be sure to get out there and spend some time playing in it! You are never too old to play in the snow. (Just don't fall and get hurt!)

January 22

Do you ever get lonesome?

Our world has become a very lonely place. You can be completely surrounded by people and yet feel utterly lonely. Utterly invisible.

Do you ever feel lonely? How do you combat it?

Meditate on what loneliness means to you. How can you better equip yourself to deal with any loneliness you may feel? More importantly, how can you prevent it in the first place?

January 23

Season of stillness

Perform this meditation in a safe place outside as early in the morning or as late at night as you can.

While we consider winter the season of stillness, not everything stops. Spend time in meditation simply listening to the stillness around you. What sounds stick out? How does the stillness, or even lack thereof, differ from other seasons? Can you feel a difference? Connect with your environment, acknowledging what you hear. Depending on where you live, there may be noticeable stillness, while other locations, not so much. Compare what you experience to other seasons where you live or compare them to other places you have lived. How do the differences affect you?

January 24

Smoke the herb: thyme

Thyme is associated with good health and courage. This has a wonderful savory scent and taste and can intensify your high.

Combine your cannabis with some dried ground thyme. I use a mix of about 80 percent cannabis to 20 percent thyme, but you can adjust that according to your preferences.

When combining herbs with cannabis for the first time, always resort back to "slow and low." You are introducing a new combination of acids, proteins, and terpenes to your system. Give yourself time to see how it affects you, and that's all you have to do. Meditate on your reactions: how does it make you feel? Do you like it? How can you use this combination further in your practices?

January 25

Opportunities

In order to get what we want, we have to not only seize opportunities given to us, we have to create our own.

What opportunities have you passed on? What were the results or ramifications of passing on those opportunities?

What opportunities have you created for yourself? How did those work out for you?

What opportunities can you create for yourself now? How do you plan to ensure their success?

January 26
Set your sights
Even though the dark half of the year is focused on inner workings, don't lose sight of what your goals are for the year. Look ahead at what you want to accomplish in the coming year. What does the completion of your goals look like? How does it make you feel to see yourself succeed? Keep this picture in your mind as you work towards achieving your goals this year.

January 27
Rest and recuperation
How often do you take time for real rest and recuperation? Meditate about it. Do you do enough of it? Are you constantly stressed? Do you need to force yourself into rest? On the opposite side, do you spend too much time resting and not enough building and expending energy? Rest and recuperation need to be balanced parts of our lives. Rest helps keep us healthy both physically and mentally. Evaluate your current practices; do you need to make changes? If so, what are they and how will you incorporate them?

January 28
Breathe it in: eucalyptus oil
Eucalyptus oil is used for healing, purification, and protection.

Decide how you want to work with the oil in a physical sense and prepare your meditation area ahead of time. For example, you may want to use a diffuser to which you can add a few drops of oil or use a self-lighting charcoal tablet in a fireproof container. Once the tablet is lit, add a few drops of oil to it for an intense burst of the scent. If you want to use the oil on your skin, be sure to add it to a carrier oil first. Never apply an essential oil directly to your skin, it can result in burns, allergic reactions, or other irritations. To keep it simple, sniff the oil from the bottle.

Next, focus on your intention for using this oil. Do you need some healing in your life? Would you like to cleanse and purify your aura? Do you want to add a protective layer around you?

Close your eyes and inhale the scent deeply and slowly several times before allowing yourself to breathe normally again. Immerse yourself in the scent so that you feel its presence all around you. If you need to, take more slow, deep breaths to increase the intensity of the scent. Focus on your intention while inhaling the scent. Envision your intention coming to fruition in your mind's eye. You are healing. Your aura is being cleansed. A protective layer is enveloping you.

Feel free to add music to this meditation.

January 29
Trance dance

For this month's trance dance, pick a song that isn't too fast, one that allows you to move freely, ethereally yet intentionally. Let it be a song that invokes the feel of a long, pleasant journey ahead of you. It is the beginning of the journey of the calendar year. Choose a song that represents this journey for you.

I use "Shamanic Journey (Om Shanti)" by Anugama.

When you are ready, begin moving with the music. Block out everything but the sound of the music.

If physical limitations require it, remain seated while moving to the music.

You can "dance" with whatever body parts you want to use. Feel free to move in whatever way feels the most pleasing to you.

Allow the music to wash over and consume you.

Where does it take you?

January 30
Create order

Order and balance are essential to keep our lives healthy and functioning. Order can be needed both internally and externally.

Use your meditation time to evaluate the order in your life. Are there changes you can make to help your life run more smoothly?

January 31
Breathwork

End your month with some good deep grounding breathwork.

Begin by inhaling, holding, and exhaling for a count of five. After three rounds, increase to a count of six.

After another three rounds, increase to a count of seven. Continue adding on to your count after every three rounds until you hit a good, deep, comfortable level. Continue to breathe this way for several minutes.

Feel yourself connecting with the earth below you with each breath.

While you breathe, think back over the past month. This month you have been working on inner parts of yourself. Which meditations have helped you the most? While we are still in the dead of winter—the time of rest and recuperation—the new calendar year has started. Evaluate what you have accomplished so far if you have set goals to achieve.

✳ FEBRUARY SHOPPING LIST ✳

Amethyst (February 9)

Dried crushed rose petals (February 12)

3 chocolate truffles all different flavors (February 14)

Rose essential oil (February 20)

February 1
Inspiration and creativity

There is no doubt that weed is great for jumpstarting inspiration and creativity. Cannabis has literally been used for thousands of years for just this reason. Allow your journey today to explore what inspires you. Let your creativity flow, and allow your meditation to take you wherever it wants to go.

February 2
Awaken

As the year passes on, the energies begin to shift. Nature finds itself beginning the switch from slumber to awakening. Below the frozen ground in the north, life is preparing for the journey forward. Over the dark half of the year, you have worked internally. The shift to the external and to new life is now beginning.

Meditate on what awakening means to you. Do you feel the awakening in nature around you?

February 3
Cleansing release

Internal work can bring up mixed emotions, stressful memories, and bad experiences. A cleansing release helps you to wash away clinging negativities. Use this meditation to visualize your spirit being cleansed. You may want to imagine a bright light or even a beautiful waterfall washing over you. Fit your cleansing to what works best for you. Spend as much time as you like in your meditation, feeling yourself releasing anything that no longer serves you. Allow your spirit to be fully cleansed.

February 4
Feel the goodness

Today is about positivity and just feeling the goodness all around you. Meditate on all of the good things you have going on in your life. Revel in that goodness. Feel the joy it brings you. Experience the gratitude you feel for having so much that is good in your life.

February 5
Quiet time

Today we are constantly bombarded with stimulation from social media, TV, other people. It gets to be too much. This constant stimulation can cause anxiety, sleep issues, and a variety of mental and physical health issues. Meditation is an excellent way to combat these stimuli.

Spend today's meditation in simple quiet time; allow your brain to relax. Daydream, zone out, or chill, but if you catch yourself thinking about current events or worrying about something you need to do, redirect your mind. Tell your brain not now. Take your mind to a happy, relaxed, location. No stress. No worries. No concerns or stimulus. Simply peace and quiet reserved for you.

February 6
Reflection
Now that we are a month into the new calendar year, take some time today to reflect on how things are going for you so far. Have you started working towards any of your goals? Evaluate where you are at and compare to your expectations. You don't need to judge or chastise yourself if you aren't where you expected. Simply acknowledge where you are now and reflect on what you have accomplished so far.

February 7
Holding uncertainty
Uncertainty can be frustrating. It can be scary. It can also be a blessing in disguise. Uncertainty tells us patience is needed before a decision should be made. Uncertainty

tells us the future is in motion and that multiple outcomes are possible. Uncertainty tells us we have a chance to make a change for the better.

How does being uncertain about something make you feel? Do you fear the uncertain? Do you embrace it? Meditate on what it means to you and how you can use uncertainty to your advantage in the future.

February 8
Clarity

People often claim one of the downsides of cannabis use is that it clouds the mind. What they do not realize is that in the proper dosage, it gives the user an extreme amount of clarity. Since everyone's dosage is different, you need to experiment to find what works best for you.

Today, focus on a situation that you have issues comprehending. Try seeing the situation from different angles and different points of view.

Allow the cannabis to do its job and help open your eyes to these other viewpoints. You don't have to be happy with the situation or agree to it, but understanding and receiving clarity on the situation does give you the needed information to be able to deal with it in a way that will be most beneficial to you.

See the situation for what it is, taking in all the information you can. Use this clarity to find the most appropriate path.

February 9

Get stoned: amethyst

Amethyst is a purple stone that resonates with wisdom, courage, healing addictions, peace, love, happiness, psychic energy, and dreams.

Pick one of these qualities that calls to you. What do you need to call into your life? Get into your comfy spot and hold the stone in your hand out in front of you.

Examine the stone with your eyes and your fingers.

Feel the stone as you hold it tightly in your hand.

Hold the stone close to your heart.

Meditate on the stone and how it feels to you.

Feel a connection with the stone. Charge your stone by imagining it filled with that quality you seek.

Do you need a bit of courage? Whether it be in speaking up for yourself or others, amethyst has your back. Issues with an addiction? Charge your amethyst to help heal your addictions. Give yourself the gift of peace, love, and happiness with a triple-charged stone.

Feel the attribute you want to work with present in your stone.

Carry this stone with you whenever you feel the need.

February 10
Call of the wild: snowfall sounds
Do an online search for "snowfall sounds."

Find a clip that is a good length for your meditation time or use the repeat feature.

Play the clip and meditate on it as you listen.

Do you like this sound? Dislike the sound?

Let the sound encompass you.

How does it make you feel?

February 11
Get up the nerve
You don't have to be shy to be nervous about doing something. Sometimes it can be very difficult to get up the nerve to do certain things, particularly when those "things" lead to change. Change is hard to accept, even when it's a good change. We are creatures of habit, and changing those habits can make us anxious.

Meditate on how well you are able to (or not able to) get up the nerve in different situations. What makes it difficult for you? What makes it easy? Are there motivators you can engage in the future to help you when necessary? Evaluate without judgement.

February 12

Smoke the herb: rose

Rose can be used for several different purposes. It corresponds with love, sex, beauty, peace, luck, protection, and psychic powers.

Combine your cannabis with some dried ground rose petals. Use a mix of about 80 percent cannabis to 20 percent rose petals, but you can adjust that according to your preferences.

Be sure you are using food grade rose petals. Roses bought in the store are filled with chemicals and colorings. Do not use those. You can either grow your own (and be sure not to use anything on them!) or purchase food grade.

When combining herbs with cannabis for the first time, always resort back to "slow and low." You are introducing a new combination of acids, proteins, and terpenes to your system. Give yourself time to see how it affects you, and that's all you have to do. Meditate on your reactions: How does it make you feel? Do you like it? How can you use this combination further in your practices?

February 13

Beauty inside

We live in a world that focuses on outer beauty and often forget true beauty comes from inside. When you find your own inner beauty, you can nurture it and allow it to grow for others to see through your attitude and behaviors.

Meditate on what your inner beauty is. How can you let it grow? How can you show it to other people?

February 14

Got the munchies: chocolate truffles

Today is when many celebrate love, so what better day to show yourself a little love with the truffle(s) of your choice?

After dosing, get into your comfy spot and set the truffles right by you. This meditation is going to focus on your taste buds and other sensations. Keep your eyes closed so that you are not relying on your sense of sight. When you are ready, take a bite of a truffle. Using your sense of smell, can you identify the flavor? Pay extreme attention to what you are doing. Feel your teeth sink into the truffle. Experience the textures and flavors. Singling them out as much as possible. Take your time and enjoy the truffle. When you are ready, continue with the others. Are you able to identify and distinguish the flavors from each other? Use this type of meditation anytime you are eating for a fuller, richer connection with your food.

February 15
Chill lounge

For part of the United States, February is the worst time for cold and snow. At the same time, however, the days have been growing longer and the sun begins to break through the clouds. We know that winter isn't over; the worst of things may not even be behind us yet, but we know deep down that warmer days, better days, are coming. The light at the end of the tunnel is shining brightly and coaxing us on.

Find a song that reflects this feeling, these emotions of strength and promise for you. I use "Winter's Light" by Tim Janis.

Play your music while you are in your comfy spot. Let not only the music but any lyrics flow over you, and listen deeply and intently. Where does the music take you? How does it make you feel?

February 16
Inspirational inklings

"When you smoke the herb, it reveals you to yourself."

—Bob Marley[3]

---

3. Bob Marley and Ian McCann, *Bob Marley "Talking": Bob Marley in His Own Words* (London: Omnibus Press, 2003), n.p.

Marley may never have stated truer words. Cannabis drops your walls and allows you to see yourself and your actions from an objective viewpoint. It allows you to see things you had not seen before about yourself and your situations in life. Smoke up and let the herb reveal something about yourself to you today.

February 17

Be immune

Remember the childhood saying "Sticks and stones may break my bones, but names will never hurt me"?

We told ourselves that as children, but it wasn't true.

Names did hurt.

Words did hurt.

They still can.

What we didn't know as children, though, is that bad names and words say far more about the person using them than they do about ourselves.

We can be immune when someone tries to use them against us because we now know it's not about us, it's about them.

Think back to a time when you didn't know this. Tell your younger self this tidbit of knowledge. How would knowing this sooner have changed this specific situation?

Allow yourself to heal from it now.

February 18

Your inner critic

We all have one. That nagging voice that occasionally pops up to throw us off or cause us to second guess ourselves.

What else does your inner critic tell you?

Does it show up often or seldom?

How does it make you feel when it does speak up?

Do you listen and evaluate what it has to say?

While your inner critic can have a negative connotation, learn to turn what it tells you to the positive.

February 19

Sacred dream

Your sacred dream is, simply put, the dream you hold most sacred. Realistic or not, it is a part of why you exist. When you dream about your "perfect life," what does it include? Your perfect career? Your perfect relationship? Your perfect version of yourself? If there were no limitations placed on you, what would you dream up for your life? Spend today meditating on what your sacred dream is. Add in as many details as you can. Live this dream in your meditation.

February 20

Breathe it in: rose oil

Rose oil is used for attracting love, sexual arousal, peace, luck, and beauty.

Decide your purpose for working with the oil: Are you looking to attract love? Do you already have a committed partner whose love you want to honor? Do you want to use it to bring yourself luck or peace or both? Prepare your meditation area ahead of time. You may want to use a diffuser to which you can add a few drops of oil. Use a self-lighting charcoal tablet in a fireproof container, and once the tablet is lit, add a few drops of oil to it for an intense burst of the scent. If you want to use the oil on your skin, be sure to add it to a carrier oil first. To keep it simple, sniff the oil from the bottle.

Use the oil in your chosen method. Close your eyes and inhale the scent deeply and slowly several times before allowing yourself to breathe normally again. Immerse yourself in the scent so that you feel its aura all around you. If you need to, take more slow, deep breaths to increase the intensity of the scent.

What feelings does this scent invoke in you? Does it bring back memories? Do you have a connection to this scent?

Feel free to add music to this meditation.

February 21
Soul refuge

Create in your mind your perfect refuge. Is it a real location you are familiar with or is it a self-created image? See it clearly in your mind's eye.

What do you hear?

Smell?

Feel?

Create as many details as you can. What about these details comforts you?

When you feel the need, take a moment to step into your soul asylum to refresh and rejuvenate.

You can change this refuge any time you want.

February 22
Get lost

Every now and then, we all need a little escape from life. Today, spend your meditation getting lost in some place you really wish you could be. Whether it's imaginary or real, spend your meditation lost in your chosen world. How does being here make you feel?

February 23
Trance dance

The light at the end of the tunnel is spring, and she is visible though still out of reach. The sight of her fills you with hope and the promise of things to come. Plans you have been considering, workings you have been doing over the dark half—their time will soon be expiring. The spring is coming, and with it comes a new dawn, a new beginning, a new time to let yourself shine. For now, your focus is still inward, but do enjoy an occasional glimpse into your future to come.

Find a song that gives you hope for the things to come. A song that promises new beginnings are just around the bend. The time for rest will soon be over, and the season will again turn.

I like to use "Winter" by Ryan Farish.

When you are ready, begin moving with the music. Block out everything but the sound of the music.

If physical limitations require it, remain seated while moving to the music.

You can "dance" with whatever body parts you want to use. Feel free to move in whatever way feels the most pleasing to you.

Allow the music to wash over and consume you.

Where does it take you?

February 24
Chant
"Sky above.
Earth below.
Air my life.
Fire my soul."

This is a simple chant to help you center and ground. Feel each connection as you say them. Picture the sky above. Touch the earth below. Inhale the air that brings you life. Feel the passion that fires your soul.

Repeat this chant throughout your meditation.

Try saying it in different intonations and at different speeds until you find your match.

How does this chant make you feel?

What does it mean to you?

February 25
Letting go
We carry around burdens every day that we do not need. Things from the past that creep up on us and weigh us down. Letting go can be a scary concept, but when you realize you aren't really holding on to anything, it makes it easier. The past is the past. It's over and cannot be changed. What you are holding on to doesn't exist anymore. Let it go. Spend your meditation saying goodbye to

a burden that has been holding you down. Let it fly free and remove the weight from your soul.

February 26

I forgive you

Forgiveness is a key to moving on in life. When we forgive others, we also lift a burden and weight off our own shoulders.

Who do you need to forgive? Without rehashing the situation, think about who has harmed you. Do you know what their intention was? Did they mean harm or was it an unfortunate side effect?

Whether the other person ever knows if you forgive them or not, you need to forgive them in your own heart and let their offense go.

You cannot choose how other people act, but you can choose how you react to them.

Meditate on giving the person forgiveness. What does forgiveness look like in your situation?

Can or should the relationship be mended?

Mend yourself by offering up forgiveness in your meditation.

If possible, offer it in the mundane world.

The person may or may not want forgiveness, but your conscience will be clear.

February 27
Inspirational inklings

"Logic will get you from A to B. Imagination will take you everywhere."

—Albert Einstein[4]

Sometimes we get so caught up in life dealing with the details—work, bills, family, other commitments—we forget to use our imaginations. As children, we use our imaginations frequently, but the older we get, many of us simply stop. Use your imagination today and let it take you anywhere.

February 28
Breathwork

End your month with some grounding and reflective breathwork.

Begin by inhaling, holding, and exhaling for a count of five. After three rounds, increase to a count of six.

After another three rounds, increase to a count of seven. Continue adding on to your count after every three rounds until you hit a good, deep, comfortable level. Continue to breathe this way for several minutes.

---

4. Alice Calaprice, *The Ultimate Quotable Einstein* (Princeton, NJ: Princeton University Press, 2011), 481.

Pick a moment from the past month that was particularly happy or helpful for you. Hold that moment and reflect upon it. We often focus on the negative times we have. Change that habit and hold on to the good instead. Spend as much time in your joy as you like.

February 29
Take a leap

What is something you have always wanted to do but for one reason or another you just haven't done it?

Maybe you are afraid or nervous it won't work out right or you will fail.

But you can't succeed if you never try.

Today, meditate on what leap you want to take.

What is the worst thing that can happen? What is the best?

Come up with a plan of action and then implement it.

✷ MARCH SHOPPING LIST ✷

Aquamarine (March 9)

Myrrh essential oil (March 14)

Dried crushed raspberry leaf (March 18)

Fresh pineapple chunks (March 25)

March 1
Inspirational inklings

"All true artists, whether they know it or not, create from a place of no-mind, from inner stillness."

—Eckhart Tolle[5]

Sit back and relax. Focus on your own inner stillness. Let your mind go as blank as it wants and rest there for a bit. Let what wants to emerge do so. What can you create?

March 2
Inner peace

Today's meditation is simple and relaxing. Find your inner peace. Imagine yourself enveloped in a loving hug from yourself or from someone that makes you feel calm and at peace. Perhaps a child, a spouse, or your deity. Feel

---

5. Eckhart Tolle, *The Power of Now: A Guide to Spiritual Enlightenment* (Hachette Australia, 2018), 17.

yourself safe and relaxed. Allow your mind to take you to where it needs to go.

March 3
New beginnings

Spring is officially just days away. The earth is awakening and beginning anew.

What new beginnings do you have planned for your life? Choose one or two of them to focus on for this meditation.

Meditate on the new beginning you have planned. Imagine all the details you can, and imagine where this new beginning will take you. See everything in a positive light. Do not let the thought of failure or things not working out right enter your mind. Only positives. See your new beginning through to a positive fruition.

March 4
Free spirit

Today, let your spirit soar wherever your meditation wants to take you. Fly through the sky, travel across the world, visit a mythical location. Let your spirit be free and take you wherever it wants to go.

March 5
Embracing change

Most of us have been programmed to associate change with some type of negativity, but we can adjust our views on change by erasing the negative connotation. Embrace change. Know that change opens the door for new possibilities and new relationships.

Stop looking at change as an ending. Look at it as a new beginning instead.

What changes have you had a hard time with lately? Have you looked at change as a negative or positive? How can you reframe your thoughts to shift them from a negative outlook to a more positive one?

March 6
Inspirational inklings

"I have always loved marijuana. It has been a source of joy and comfort to me for many years. And I still think of it as a basic staple of life, along with beer and ice and grapefruits—and millions of Americans agree with me."

—Hunter S. Thompson[6]

---

6. "Hunter S Thompson: In His Own Words," *The Guardian*, February 21, 2005, https://www.theguardian.com/books/2005/feb/21/hunters thompson.

What joy and comfort has cannabis brought to you? Is it a basic staple of life for you?

March 7
Sustainably sourced

"Sustainably sourced" is an incredibly popular term in today's world. Simply put, it means to use something at a rate where consumption will not exceed production. While it generally refers to natural resources such as trees, oil, or fish, we would all be better off if we realized we ourselves should also be sustainably sourced.

You are a natural resource. Your energy is a natural resource, and as such, it needs time to replenish itself.

Without the proper ingredients and processes, it is difficult to replenish your energy.

Evaluate how well your energy is sustainably sourced. Do you eat the way you should? What are your sleep habits like? Are you able to wake up in the morning feeling refreshed and ready to go or are you dragging and barely able to open your eyes? What do you do well? Where do you have room for improvement?

March 8
Spring cleaning

Spring is almost officially here and it's time to start the spring cleaning process. Throw out the old and make way for the new. This isn't just for material possessions, but for attitudes, beliefs, habits, even relationships. What do you have in your life that no longer serves your purpose? What can you "clean out" to make room for something new? Meditate today on what you can, and should, clean out of your life.

March 9

Get stoned: aquamarine

Aquamarine is a light blue stone that resonates with serenity, peace, self-expression, purification, and psychic awareness.

Pick one of these qualities that calls to you. What do you need to call into your life? Get into your comfy spot and hold the stone in your hand out in front of you.

Examine the stone with your eyes and your fingers.

Feel the stone as you hold it tightly in your hand.

Hold the stone close to your heart.

Meditate on the stone and how it feels to you.

Feel a connection with the stone. Charge your stone by imagining it filled with that quality you seek.

Do you have a stressful week up ahead? Charge your aquamarine with serenity and peace. Do you need to find a creative outlet? Do you have issues speaking your mind? Charge your stone with self-expression. Charge an aquamarine with purification to drop into your bathtub for a cleansing bath. Do you work with divination? Dream analysis? Or do you need a bit of insight into how your boss is thinking? Charge your stone with psychic awareness.

Feel the attribute you want to work with present in your stone.

Carry this stone with you whenever you feel the need.

March 10
Call of the wild: rain sounds

Do an online search for "rain sounds."

Find a rain sounds video or audio clip that is a good length for your meditation time or use a repeat feature.

Play the clip and meditate on it as you listen.

Do you like this sound? Dislike the sound?

Let the sound encompass you.

How does it make you feel?

March 11
Spread your wings

Have fun with this peaceful yet energizing meditation.

As spring inches closer and closer, it's time to spread your wings, flap them out to shake off the dust, give them a good long stretch, and get ready to fly. Before liftoff, take in your surroundings, check for conditions, watch for possible hazards, and then take flight.

Are you a bird?

A butterfly?
A dragon?
Spread your wings and soar.

March 12
On the spiritual path

During today's meditation, evaluate the spiritual path you have been traveling on. How has it twisted and turned? How has it nourished you to grow? How has cannabis contributed to your spiritual journey? What were your high (no pun intended) moments? What were your lows? Look back on your path so far and give thanks for all that it has been—both good and bad.

March 13
If I don't do anything to make it better, who will?

This is a question we all need to start asking ourselves more often. How often do you complain about something? How often do you wish things were different in your town? School? Job? Home?

Self-responsibility seems to be lacking in today's society, and we all need to step up. But don't wait for others around you to step up before you decide to. Be the first. Make the changes you want and need in your life.

What can you do in your life now, in your environment, to make things better?

March 14

Breathe it in: myrrh oil

Myrrh oil is used for healing, protection, transformation, concentration, meditation, and spirituality.

Decide your purpose for working with the oil. Do you have healing to do—whether emotional or physical? Are you going through a transformation? Myrrh is good to encourage a meditative and spiritual state. Choose what correspondence(s) you want to focus on for this session.

Prepare your meditation area ahead of time. You may want to use a diffuser to which you can add a few drops of oil. Use a self-lighting charcoal tablet in a fireproof container, and once the tablet is lit, add a few drops of oil to it for an intense burst of the scent. If you want to use the oil on your skin, be sure to add it to a carrier oil first. To keep it simple, sniff the oil from the bottle.

Use the oil in your chosen method. Close your eyes and inhale the scent deeply and slowly several times before allowing yourself to breathe normally again. Immerse yourself in the scent so that you feel its aura all around you. If you need to, take more slow, deep breaths to increase the intensity of the scent.

What feelings does this scent invoke in you? Does it bring back memories? Do you have a connection to this scent?

Feel free to add music to this meditation.

March 15
The time is now
Meditation is the perfect way to spend time in the moment. In the present. Spend today's meditation in the now. See yourself in this moment only, no past, no future, no problems, no worries, just enjoy sitting, relaxing, and breathing in the now. Feel yourself alive, vibrant, fully present and completely aware of your surroundings. Allow being in the now to relax and rejuvenate your body and mind.

March 16
Chill lounge
By now, daylight has grown noticeably longer than it was just a month ago. The sun comes out more often. Snow is melting. Ice is thawing. Springs are flowing once again. Our energy, which has been turned inward, may begin to feel stagnant. It wants to move. It wants to turn outward and grow like the crocus bursting through the ground. It is a time of change. A time of enlightening. A time to shift your focus from the inward to the outward.

Choose a song that fills these emotions for you. I use "Spring" by Patrick Kelly.

Play your music while you are in your comfy spot. Let not only the music but any lyrics flow over you, and listen deeply and intently. Where does the music take you? How does it make you feel?

March 17

Go with the green

Before today's meditation, look up images of the Irish countryside. With the lush greens throughout the land, there is no doubt as to why it is called the Emerald Isle.

In America, regardless of their religion or heritage, many people love to celebrate the Irish on St. Patrick's Day, often by dressing in green and drinking to excessive amounts. However, Ireland itself had quite a different take on St. Patrick's Day until the past few decades. For the Irish it is a far more somber, religious holiday that, until the 1970s, pubs actually closed for. Yes—Irish pubs used to be closed on St. Patrick's Day. In the 90s the government began hosting St. Patrick's Day festivities in Dublin to encourage tourism. Today, you will find both types of celebrations—those people who will be at parades and festivals throughout the country and those who will be in church.

Let today's meditation take you to the Emerald Isle. Immerse yourself in the images you saw. Travel back in time inside your mind. What would life have been like in the fifth century when Patrick was in Ireland?

March 18

Smoke the herb: raspberry leaf

Raspberry leaf is used metaphysically to attract and keep love in your life. It is also used for fidelity and faithfulness.

Combine your cannabis with some dried, ground, organic, food grade raspberry leaf. Use a mix of about 80 percent cannabis to 20 percent raspberry leaf, but you can adjust that according to your preferences.

When combining herbs with cannabis for the first time, always resort back to "slow and low." You are introducing a new combination of acids, proteins, and terpenes to your system. Give yourself time to see how it affects you, and that's all you have to do. Meditate on your reactions: How does it make you feel? Do you like it? How can you use this combination further in your practices?

March 19

Dream weaver

There are many theories of what dreams are, with the scientific world and metaphysical world offering different opinions.

On the metaphysical side, dreams may be memories, messages from the gods or our higher selves, or even premonitions.

Learning to listen to, or how to analyze, your dreams is often a beneficial skill to have.

Spend today's meditation reviewing any recent dreams you have had. Are they somehow connected? What kind of symbolism was present? What purposes have your dreams served you?

March 20
Find your balance
Life is hectic. There are always things to be done, places to go, people to see. How do you find balance in your life?

Does your life feel out of whack? Do you spend time working on your physical, mental, emotional, and spiritual health? Do you do more for others than you do for yourself? Do you do more for yourself than you do for others?

Spend time in meditation evaluating where you land on the scale. Is your life in balance? If not, what changes do you need to make to adjust it? If you are in balance, reflect on your journey to get there.

March 21
Make a seasonal offering
Start the new season off with an offering. It does not have to be a physical offering, but an offering from your heart, mind, or spirit. Give this offering to your deities, your higher power, or the universe at large.

It can be an emotion or feeling you offer up such as "peace for all mankind." It can be a special prayer.

You can make it a physical offering tied into the season—while doing spring cleaning, gather items to donate to a local charity. You can also volunteer to help with other spring cleaning. Many parks, townships, cities, and forest preserves need volunteers to help with garbage pickup in parks and along roadways. Elderly or other invalids may need help with spring cleaning too, especially yard work and gutter cleaning.

Meditate on what offerings you have to give.

March 22
Renewal

Spring is all about renewal, rebirth, and rejuvenation.

Renewal gives us a fresh start, a fresh outlook on life or whatever situation you are dealing with. Renewal is a new start, a new beginning, a chance to change things that haven't worked well in the past, and an opportunity to try something new for the future.

What areas of your life need a fresh start? A clean slate to restart from?

Meditate today on what has not been working for you and how you can adjust your outlook and actions to give yourself a new start.

March 23

Transformation

Transformation is defined as a change in form, appearance, nature, or character. Spring is filled with transformations in nature all around us. We see it as the buds begin to swell on trees. Plants have begun bursting green shoots through the ground. Everything around you is coming alive once again. It is time for you to transform. All winter long, you have worked on your internal self. It is time for us to emerge from the dark half of the year and into the light, and to ensure what you have learned about yourself is put into practice and everyday use. This is how we grow and flourish, by transforming ourselves into more loving, kind, and enlightened people. Envision yourself stepping out of the darkness and into the light. Stretch as if waking from a long winter's nap. Feel the sunlight of the light half of the year on your skin, warming you.

How have you grown? What have you learned? How have you transformed?

March 24

A different perspective

Two people can look at a situation and have totally different perspectives on what they have seen. Unfortunately, this often leads to disagreements that affect relationships.

Meditate on a recent disagreement you had. Now that you have had some time to process the situation, are you able to see the other person's view? Could you see it at the time? Did you even want to see it at the time?

In the heat of an argument, we often don't want to see things from any other point of view. Evaluate how well you are able to do this. What can you do differently in the future if you need to improve in this area?

March 25

Got the munchies: pineapple

Prepare a bowl of bite-sized pineapple chunks.

After dosing, get into your comfy spot and set the pineapple right by you. This meditation is going to focus on your taste buds and other sensations. Keep your eyes closed so that you are not relying on your sense of sight. Use your sense of smell to take in the scent of the pineapple. Pay extreme attention to what you are doing as you take a bite. Feel your teeth sink into the pineapple. Experience the textures and flavor, singling them out as much as possible. Take your time and enjoy the pineapple. Use this type of meditation anytime you are eating for a fuller, richer connection with your food.

March 26
Inspiration

What inspires you? You probably get inspiration from many different areas in your life, but what about those inspirations speak to you deep down inside? Analyze the different aspects of inspiration you seek in your life. What do they say to you? What commonalities do they have? Differences? What speaks to you?

March 27
Trance dance

Connecting with the universe in dance is an age-old ritual dating back thousands of years the world over. Choose a slower song to work with while connecting to the universe in your trance dance. Be sure you have plenty of space to move as you may often lose your place and awareness of your surroundings when dancing in this manner and a full uninhibited connection is made. Pick a song that invites you to connect with the universe.

I love "Dance of Shiva" by KarmaCosmic.

When you are ready, begin moving with the music. Block out everything but the sound of the music.

If physical limitations require it, remain seated while moving to the music.

You can "dance" with whatever body parts you want to use. Feel free to move in whatever way feels the most pleasing to you.

Allow the music to wash over and consume you.

Where does it take you?

March 28

Unity

The state of oneness—the moment when you can feel yourself in such complete sync with the universe or your deity, you cannot tell where one begins and the other ends.

Finding unity with the universe is the goal of a peak experience. While it's not always possible or necessary to hit a peak experience while meditating, it does open a whole new level of understanding for the user when they do hit it.

You know you have hit a peak experience when you feel completely at one with the universe or divinity.

Try to hit a peak today and experience the feeling of unity. Even if you don't hit a peak, allow your boundaries and your perception of your physical body to blur. This blurring helps to open the door to experience true unity with the universe.

Focus on bringing down any walls you have, relax, and let the cannabis guide you on your way.

March 29
Chant
"Spring has come.
Winter is done.
Life to emerge
and welcome the sun."

This is a fun, energy-building chant to help raise your spirits and to welcome the new life brought by the spring.

Repeat this chant throughout your meditation.

Try saying it in different intonations and at different speeds until you find your match.

How does this chant make you feel?

What does it mean to you?

March 30
Change your life
One small change in your life can make a world of difference later down the road. Some changes are difficult, but there are many simple changes you can make that have positive effects. Maybe you still haven't learned to turn off the water while brushing your teeth. Maybe you want to commit to smiling more. Make eye contact with more people. Start saving five dollars a week. Drink less caffeine. Drink more water. Whatever it is, meditate today on one small change you can make, and then make it.

March 31

Breathwork

End your month with rejuvenating breathwork.

Begin by inhaling, holding, and exhaling for a count of five. After three rounds, increase to a count of six. Continue to breathe this way for several minutes.

March is about rebirth, the beginning of spring, life starting over. Our goals we planned over the dark half of the year should now be in action.

Feel the hope, the energy, the potential in your life and soul.

Anticipate happiness and success.

✳ APRIL SHOPPING LIST ✳

Quartz (April 9)

Fresh mango chucks (April 21)

Ginger essential oil (April 25)

Dried crushed hyssop (April 27)

April 1
April Fool's Day

Known as the day of fools, people use this day to pull pranks on each other.

The Fool card from the Major Arcana in tarot decks takes a different approach to what the fool symbolizes.

The Fool is on a journey and needs to pay attention to where he is going; there are dangers and pitfalls all around him, but there are also great wonders that can be easily distracting. Stay the course and stay on your path.

Meditate today on the path you are taking. What pitfalls have you tumbled into? Which ones did you spot ahead of time and successfully dodged? What great wonders have distracted your course? If you have strayed from your path, how can you work your way back to it?

April 2
Reflection

Take some time today to reflect on how things are going for you so far this year. Have you started working towards any of your goals? Evaluate where you are at and compare to your expectations. You don't need to judge or chastise yourself if you aren't where you expected. Simply acknowledge where you are now and reflect on what you have accomplished so far.

April 3
The question to ask

"How are you?" is a common overused greeting which, honestly, most people really do not want to know the answer to. Instead of this trite drivel, incorporate a new question to ask, but ask it of yourself first in today's meditation. The question is "Are you happy?" Spend today's meditation thinking about this. How happy are you with your life? Have you been working on the things you want to accomplish? Have you been putting things aside and forgetting about them? What does true happiness look like to you? What does it incorporate? When you are ready, start greeting the people you know and care for with this simple, yet thought-provoking question.

April 4

Divine intervention

Whether you work with deity, spirits, the universe, or your own higher power, we all have that little voice in our head that pops in for occasional visits. Sometimes it's to tell us "No, don't do that" or "This doesn't feel right" or some other warning not to proceed on the present course of action. Do you listen to that little voice? Do you hush it or ignore it? How has listening (or not listening) worked out for you? Have you had moments when you didn't listen but wish you had? Meditate today on how that little voice has served you in the past. How can you ensure a better relationship with that little voice in the future?

April 5

Inspirational inklings

"When I was a kid…I inhaled frequently. That was the point."

— Barack Obama, *44th President of the United States*[7]

President Obama was open about his cannabis use and even wrote about it in his 1995 memoir *Dreams from My Father.*

---

7. Holden Blunts, *The Quotable Stoner: More Than 1,100 Baked, Lit-Up, and Zonked-Out Quotes in Tribute to (And As a Result of) Smoking Weed* (Avon, MA: Adams Media, 2011), n.p.

Meditate on this quote. How open are you about your usage? Is it well known among your family and friends that you partake in the leaf? Do you feel the need to hide it from some people? If so, why? How would your life change if you were more (or less, if the case may be) open about your usage?

April 6

April showers bring May flowers

This old saying regarding the weather has another more symbolic meaning. Sometimes we may have to suffer a bit before things get better.

Meditate today on a time in the past where rain has fallen into your life, but when the "sun" came back out, life got better. How did you feel? Did you feel hopeless as the "rain" fell? Or did you hold on to the promise of the "sun" coming out to help grow your beautiful flowers?

Holding a positive attitude during life's toughest moments may be just what you need to get through the storm to see the benefits on the other side.

Hold on to the flowers and know that the rain always passes.

April 7

Treasures

When we are children, we have plenty of little treasures. Whether it's a special toy or a rock we happened to find on the ground, we claim them to be treasures and do not want anyone else to touch them.

As we grow older, we realize that treasures are not material objects at all. They are the people we love. They are the adventures we experience. They are the memories we cherish. These are the true treasures in the world.

Spend today's meditation focusing on your hoard. What treasures have you accumulated over the years?

April 8

Ask for what you want

Children know how to ask for what they want. Not only do they ask (a lot), they frequently demand an answer and don't give up until they get one. They end up driving their parents batty, and sometimes there are negative repercussions. Perhaps that is why when some people get older, they find it extremely difficult to ask for they want.

If you don't ever ask, though, you can't realistically expect to ever receive.

Ask the universe today in your meditation for what it is you want. Use details. Be demanding if you want. Whatever you do, let the universe know what it is you want. Ask.

April 9

Get stoned: quartz

Quartz is a clear crystal that resonates with strength, protection, healing, physical energy, psychic energy, and purification.

Choose one or more of these qualities that calls to you. What do you need to call into your life? Has your energy been low? Could you use a boost of strength and healing? Traveling and want some protection?

Get into your comfy spot and hold the stone in your hand out in front of you.

Examine the stone with your eyes and your fingers.

Feel the stone as you hold it tightly in your hand.

Hold the stone close to your heart.

Meditate on the stone and how it feels to you.

Feel a connection with the stone. Charge your stone by imagining it filled with the qualities you seek. Visualize each of these different qualities as a different colored light, swirling, filling the quartz. As they swirl and combine together, they shift into the clearness of the stone. Feel each attribute you want to work with present in your stone.

Quartz is very versatile and powerful. Fill it with all of the above intentions and you can use it as your "go to" crystal.

Carry this stone with you whenever you feel the need.

April 10

Call of the wild: thunderstorms

Do an online search for "thunderstorm sounds."

Find a thunderstorm track that is a good length for your meditation time or use the repeat feature.

Play the track and meditate on it as you listen.

Do you like this sound? Dislike the sound?

Let the sound encompass you.

How does it make you feel?

April 11

Walk away from unhealthy relationships

Relationships can really suck. They can be great, of course, but they can also really suck. There are plenty of different types of relationships that can all be boiled down to one word: unhealthy. Add to this that people only change when they want to, and you have probably found yourself in the situation of having unhealthy relationships at one time or another. Some of these relationships are far more difficult to let go than others. Invested time, relationship status (married, blood, friendship, etc.), and self-worth are all factors that contribute to the ease or difficulty in letting these relationships go. You are not only letting go of the person, you also need to let go of what you had hoped the relationship would be. This can be gut wrenching and heart breaking.

What unhealthy relationships do you have? Have you walked away from any before? Are you in the process of walking away now?

It is important to remember, and to tell ourselves when necessary, that we deserve better. We do not deserve to be walked on, abused, dismissed, or any number of other negative actions unhealthy relationships are littered with.

Tell yourself.

You deserve better.

April 12

Harmony

In music, the harmony complements the melody. It isn't the main focus, but it does add beauty to the melody by enhancing it.

What plays the role of harmony in your life? It's not your main focus, but things that add beauty to your own melody?

Meditate today on your own harmony: Is it lacking? Does it try to take over your melody? Evaluate your life song. Does it need some new chords?

April 13

Fluidity

Fluidity is an object's ability to "go with the flow." In today's meditation, use your own fluidity and let your mind go with the flow. Let it take you to wherever it wants to go. It may have a message for you or it may just want to chill. Sit back, relax, and let it flow.

April 14
Inner truth
The world is a judgmental place. What people think they know and what they truly know about others, are two very different things. Remind yourself that only you know your inner truth. Only you need to know your inner truth. You do not need acceptance or permission to be the person you want to be. All you need is your inner truth and your own desire to be who you want to be. Who does your inner truth say you are?

April 15
Determination
The drive to get what we want is tied directly to how much we want something. People who claim they have no determination have not yet found something they want badly enough to overcome obstacles to achieve it. (Why they haven't found something yet is a completely different story.) Do you find you have an abundance of drive or a lack of drive? What is it that drives you? What is it you want enough to fight for it?

April 16
Chill lounge

April weather can bring destructive thunderstorms and devastating tornadoes. Floods can wash away cars, homes, and people. The same water that gives us life can also destroy lives. But once the water recedes, and cleanup is done, life finds a way to continue again, reclaiming lost ground. Nature shares important lessons with us, even when she is destructive.

Find a song that reminds you that life goes on, even after a destructive storm.

I use "Nature's Altar" by Peter Gundry.

Play your music while you are in your comfy spot. Let not only the music but any lyrics flow over you, and listen deeply and intently. Where does the music take you? How does it make you feel?

April 17
Solitude

Solitude is often underrated. We all need it. We need to take time for ourselves to be by ourselves. Time without anyone or anything to distract from some quality alone time. Use your meditation today as a time of solitude. A time to be at peace and simply to reset. No other worries, nothing to think about or deal with. Just relax and enjoy being with yourself and only yourself.

April 18
Ebb and flow

Ebb and flow is the rhythmical pattern of coming and going or deterioration and regrowth. It's a continuous motion of alternating between two opposites. It is a part of life. Nature shows this in tides, with the changes in seasons of the year, and even in more destructive occurrences such as damaging storms, wildfires, and other natural disasters. What is grown can de destroyed and either grown again, or something new grows in its place. What patterns of ebb and flow do you have in your life? Where do you plunge forward and then retreat? Where do you find destruction and reconstruction?

April 19
Illusion

An illusion is defined as something that deceives by producing a fake impression of reality.

Sometimes, being deceived is a good thing.

Let today's meditation take you into a world of illusions. Nothing you will see is real, so why not picture some different and fun, interesting things? What can you create with your imagination?

April 20

Happy 4/20!

Today is about celebrating and honoring the herb.

Your meditation today should be just that—celebrate, honor, thank, whatever it is you need to do to express your love for and relationship with cannabis.

April 21

Got the munchies: mango

Prepare a bowl of bite-sized mango chunks.

After dosing, get into your comfy spot and set the mango right by you. This meditation is going to focus on your taste buds and other sensations. Keep your eyes closed so that you are not relying on your sense of sight. Use your sense of smell to take in the scent of the mango. Pay extreme attention to what you are doing as you take a bite. Feel your teeth sink into the mango. Experience the textures and flavor, singling them out as much as possible. Take your time and enjoy the mango. Use this type of meditation anytime you are eating for a fuller, richer connection with your food.

Mango also has the added benefit of increasing the effects of THC due to the high level of myrcene in them. Myrcene is a terpene that allows the body to absorb THC quicker and will hold your high longer by increasing the

CB1 receptor saturation level. Basically, the receptor can hold more THC.

Bay leaves, eucalyptus, hops, and lemongrass are all high in myrcene.

April 22
Change your mind

Remember the first time you realized you held a belief different from what your parents or guardians wanted you to believe? We are raised to hold certain beliefs as truth and sometimes, as we grow, we realize those beliefs don't fit in with our own personal code. It's never too late to change your mind about what you believe in. Your beliefs will change and adjust as you grow and as you gain wisdom. This is the way of life.

What beliefs have you had that have changed over your life? How has changing your beliefs changed your life?

April 23
Thank you, Mother Earth

The earth is our mother. She provides us with all the essentials for life. Food, water, air, shelter. Too often we have taken these things for granted. As more and more people stand up and defend our Mother Earth, more people learn about not only the damage we have done, but ways we can help save her. Even individuals can make a difference on how we treat our earth mother—by their actions and with their vote.

Use today's meditation to connect with and thank Mother Earth for all that she gives. Send healing energies to her. Visualize clean, pollution-free air. Visualize lakes, rivers, and oceans that flow uncluttered with debris. Visualize trees and plants growing in previously devastated areas. Somewhere out there are people who will someday find ways to solve some of our worst environmental problems. Send them energy and positive vibrations. Are you one of them? What can you do in your corner of the world to save and protect Mother Earth?

April 24
Chant

"Lokah Samastah Sukhino Bhavantu." Pronunciation: Low-KAH Sah-moss-TAH Soo-kee-NO Buh-vahn-TOO

This Sanskrit prayer translates to "May all beings everywhere be happy and free, and may the thoughts, words, and actions of my own life contribute in some way to that happiness and to that freedom for all."

As you repeat this chant, focus your energies on peace, happiness, and freedom for all, yourself included.

April 25

Breathe it in: ginger oil

Ginger corresponds with success, energy, courage, power, and sex.

Decide your purpose for working with the oil. Choose what correspondence(s) you want to focus on for this session. Ginger is perfect when you need to be bold. It is great for any situation where your confidence needs a boost. Ginger says you are powerful, successful, courageous. It is also appealing if your sex life could use a pick-me-up.

Prepare your meditation area ahead of time. You may want to use a diffuser to which you can add a few drops of oil. Use a self-lighting charcoal tablet in a fireproof container, and once the tablet is lit, add a few drops of oil to it for an intense burst of the scent. If you want to use the oil on your skin, be sure to add it to a carrier oil first. To keep it simple, sniff the oil from the bottle.

Use the oil in your chosen method. Close your eyes and inhale the scent deeply and slowly several times before allowing yourself to breathe normally again. Immerse yourself in the scent so that you feel its aura all around you. If you need to, take more slow, deep breaths to increase the intensity of the scent.

What feelings does this scent invoke in you? Does it bring back memories? Do you have a connection to this scent?

Feel free to add music to this meditation.

April 26
Self-sabotage
We can be our own worst enemy if we aren't careful. The art of self-sabotage is seldom done consciously, but for some reason or another, subconsciously there may be a desire to fail. It is often ingrained in us from an early age. Meditate today on what you have done to stand in your own way. Can you think of examples of your own self-sabotage? Let the cannabis open your mind to see what you have done to damage your own success in the past. Ask it to show you why you have partaken in screwing things up for yourself. Listen and be ready for the answer.

April 27
Smoke the herb: hyssop
Hyssop corresponds with purification, protection, prosperity, and the conscious mind.

Combine your cannabis with some dried, ground, organic, food grade hyssop. Use a mix of about 80 percent cannabis to 20 percent hyssop, but you can adjust that according to your preferences.

When combining herbs with cannabis for the first time, always resort back to "slow and low." You are introducing a new combination of acids, proteins, and terpenes to your system. Give yourself time to see how it affects you, and that's all you have to do. Meditate on your reactions: how does it make you feel? Do you like it? How can you use this combination further in your practices?

April 28
Take off your hat
We wear different hats depending on the company and situation we are in. We have many roles we play for other people: friend, coworker, counselor, employee, parent, child, etc.

For today's meditation, take off all your hats. All of them. Visualize removing each hat you can think of. Who are you once you remove who you are for everyone else? Who are you for you?

April 29
Breathwork
Lie down in your comfy spot with one hand on your stomach and one on your chest. Feel both rise and fall as you inhale and exhale. Slow your breathing, drawing it

out as long as is comfortable. Focus on ridding yourself of any negative energies from the month that you have had difficulties with. Allow anything negative to flow out with your exhalation. Inhale positive energy. You may want to visualize it as a white cleansing light. As you hold your breath, the light scrubs away at any tension held in your body. Allow any negative feelings to flow outward with the release of your breath. Out with the old, in with the new. Breathe yourself into a refreshed state of body and mind.

April 30
Trance dance

The celebrations of May Day are at hand. Different countries have different traditions, but many of these traditions involve intense dancing to be performed. It is a time to raise energy, and there are few better ways than in a dance. The energy in nature is fertile and lusty. Choose a song to help you build energy and to honor the fertility of the season.

I love "Walpurgisnacht" by Faun.[8]

When you are ready, begin moving with the music. Block out everything but the sound of the music.

If physical limitations require it, remain seated while moving to the music.

You can "dance" with whatever body parts you want to use. Feel free to move in whatever way feels the most pleasing to you.

Allow the music to wash over and consume you.

Where does it take you?

---

8. Walpurgis Night is the Feast of Saint Walpurga celebrated in Germany from sunset on April 30 through sunset on May 1. Hexennacht (Witches Night) on this same date was said to be when witches met on the Brocken Mountain to wait for spring to be ushered in. Saint Walpurga was supposed to be able to repel evil sent out by the witches. In celebrations today, many Pagans have reclaimed Hexennacht and along with it, Walpurgisnacht as part of their May Day or Beltane celebrations. The song "Walpurgisnacht" by Faun is about the celebration as the witches gather together around their bonfire and dance throughout the night until the morning light.

✳ MAY SHOPPING LIST ✳

Emerald (May 13)

Dried crushed jasmine flowers (May 18)

Lilac essential oil (May 24)

Fresh apricots (May 29)

May 1
May Day

May Day, also known as Beltane, is an ancient spring holiday and festival celebrated in many parts of the Northern Hemisphere. It is a time for celebrating the return of life with dancing and other merrymaking.

Use today's meditation as part of your May Day celebration. Focus on the energy bursting forth around you as spring grows into full bloom. This is new, rejuvenated energy. Fresh and clean. Allow the energy to wash over and through you, cleansing you with renewed vitality.

May 2
Potential

You have the potential to do great things. Do you live up to it? Are you working at your highest potential? Do you give life your all or do you just try to get by? Do you push yourself or do you settle for the minimum? Evaluate how well you are living up to your own potential.

May 3

Bursting forth

Following the cycles of nature, now is the time when plants begin growing stronger. Leaves and flowers are budding and beginning to burst forth. The grass begins greening, replacing the browned death of winter. As nature focuses on her own growth and strength, so do we.

Meditate on your own growth and strength. Feel your energy building inside you—energy you pull up from your root system and push outwards, bursting forth with new life.

Celebrate this new growth.

May 4

International Star Wars Day

A day when people love to wish others "May the fourth be with you" as a play on words from the most famous line in the movies.

The Force is described as "an energy field created by all living things" by the character Obi-Wan Kenobi in *Star Wars: Episode IV—A New Hope*.

Have fun with today's meditation by visualizing the Force flowing through you and all living things. If you can, do this meditation outside to help boost your visualization technique. What does the Force feel like to you?

May 5

Vulnerability

It's difficult to admit to feeling vulnerable. We have been taught vulnerability means weakness and is an undesirable trait. We can turn this into a positive. Vulnerabilities show us where we need improvement. When a plant in the garden has vulnerabilities, we fix it. We add minerals to the soil. We use stakes to support stems so they can grow strong again. We put up fences to stop critters from eating newly grown seedlings. Doing these things allows the plants to grow and flourish and produce abundantly.

Our vulnerabilities need to be treated the same way. They are only signs of where we need help. Where we need to be nourished and protected so we, too, can grow strong and flourish.

What vulnerabilities do you see in yourself? How can you nourish and protect them so you can grow?

May 6

Phoenix rising

The phoenix dies in a burst of flames and then is reborn, rising from the ashes. It becomes a fully new creature.

Be the phoenix. Let the old you burst into flames, burning everything that no longer serves you. Habits, feelings, thoughts that are holding you back—visualize them burning into nothing but ash. See your new self as it emerges from the ash. New. Complete. Free of that which you let the fire consume.

May 7
Nourishment

Nourishment is what helps us survive. Without it, we wither and die. Food and water are nurturing to our bodies. Meditation is nurturing to your body, mind, and spirit. What other forms of nourishment do you consume? What areas of your life do they affect?

May 8
Commitment

When you make a commitment to yourself, you are not only making a promise, you are setting up a personal system of accountability. Your commitment holds you responsible to yourself. We make commitments to other people, and we stick with them, keeping our reputations intact, but will often make excuses as to why we do not keep commitments we make to ourselves. We each deserve the same respect and consideration that we give to others. We need to give this same respect and consideration to ourselves. We deserve to be treated with as much fairness as we treat others.

Make a commitment to yourself. Use your meditation to explore this promise and to pledge an oath to keep it.

May 9
Self-trust
Meditate on what self-trust issues you may have. Do you have areas you need to work on? How can you build trust with yourself?

Do you trust yourself?

Do you believe you always do the right thing?

Do you lie?

It is practically impossible to trust other people if you can't trust yourself. And if you can't trust yourself, why should anyone else trust you?

May 10
Call of the wild: bubbling brook
Do an online search for "bubbling brook sounds."

Find a bubbling brook clip that is a good length for your meditation time or use a repeat feature.

Play the song and meditate on it as you listen.

Do you like this sound? Dislike the sound?

Let the sound encompass you.

How does it make you feel?

May 11
Guidance
Seek out guidance today in your meditation. Whether it be from your deities, spirit guides, higher self, ancestors—

whomever you wish, ask for guidance. Call out in your mind to who you want to speak with. Ask them to please come to you and provide you with the assistance you seek. Visualize as they answer your call and appear to you. You may ask about a specific circumstance or just for guidance in general. What message does the universe have for you?

May 12

Reassurance

Wouldn't it be nice to have someone who can reassure you when you need it? Someone to say "You made the right choice" or "You're doing a great job at life." Someone who can reassure you that you are doing the best you can and that is all any of us can do.

You do have that someone. Yourself. Your deities. Your spirit guides. Your ancestors. Your higher power or self. All you have to do to hear them is connect with the universe and listen.

May 13

Get stoned: emerald

Emerald corresponds with astral travel, communication, courage, emotional balance, friendship, healing past life blockages, happiness, luck, prosperity, and protection.

Choose one or more of these qualities that calls to you. Emerald is another very versatile stone and can be charged with as many of these qualities as you want, or a specific one if that suits your needs better. Always ask yourself what intention the stone can help fulfill.

Get into your comfy spot and hold the stone in your hand out in front of you.

Examine the stone with your eyes and your fingers.

Feel the stone as you hold it tightly in your hand.

Hold the stone close to your heart.

Meditate on the stone and how it feels to you.

Carry this stone with you whenever you feel the need.

May 14

Inspirational inklings

"The illegality of cannabis is outrageous, an impediment to full utilization of a drug which helps produce the serenity and insight, sensitivity and fellowship so desperately needed in this increasingly mad and dangerous world."

—Carl Sagan[9]

Meditate on what Sagan says cannabis produces: serenity, insight, sensitivity, and fellowship. How can you help spread this message in our world today?

---

9. Lester Grinspoon, *Marihuana Reconsidered* (Cambridge, MA: Harvard University Press, 1977), n.p.

May 15
Stimulation

Spring is a stimulating time of year. With new life, a highly stimulating energy buzzes all around you. If possible, do today's meditation outside in nature. If you can't go outside, at least sit by an open window. It is best to do this meditation in the morning.

Visualize the energy, the life force, emanating off all the living beings around you, whether it's plants, animals, insects, pollen on the wind, or birds in the air, there is a bounty of life to be felt. Each of these living beings not only sends out but also receives energy to help them grow. The sun, earth, water, and air all fuel them. Feel the energy from the sun as it stimulates the plants to grow. See the energy as different colors, swirling and whirling in the air around you as they intermingle with each other. Invite the energy to swirl through you. Let this stimulating energy set you on an energized path for the day.

May 16
Spiritual space

Today, connect with your higher power—whether that be yourself, deity, spirit guides, the universe as a whole— whatever it is that works for you. Spend time in a spiritual space with your chosen higher power and connect. Feel the energy flow between, around, and through you.

Do you seek any assistance? Ask for help if needed. Give gratitude. Share joy.

May 17
Chill lounge

Spring is in full season. Flowers and trees bloom and leaves begin unfurling from their buds, stretching out to catch the light. The sun is bright, and the temperatures grow warmer with each day. It's time to be outside and to be active. It's time to reconnect with nature, with wildlife, with the energies of our natural world.

Choose a song that helps you connect to the energies of growth and nature.

I use "Beltane" by Narsilion.

Play your music while you are in your comfy spot. Let not only the music but any lyrics flow over you, and listen deeply and intently. Where does the music take you? How does it make you feel?

May 18
Smoke the herb: jasmine

Jasmine is a versatile herb. It corresponds with love and lust, drawing money, peace, sleep, and dreams and spirituality.

Combine your cannabis with some dried ground jasmine petals. Use a mix of about 80 percent cannabis to

20 percent jasmine, but you can adjust that according to your preferences.

When combining herbs with cannabis for the first time, always resort back to "slow and low." You are introducing a new combination of acids, proteins, and terpenes to your system. Give yourself time to see how it affects you, and that's all you have to do. Meditate on your reactions: How does it make you feel? Do you like it? How can you use this combination further in your practices?

May 19

Questioning

Weed and questioning—seriously, these two are best friends. One of the joys of cannabis is smoking a bowl, sitting around a campfire questioning the meaning of life, and, well, questioning everything. From the deep questions of "why do we exist" to the "what if there is life on other planets" to "why was Goofy able to talk and wear clothes but Pluto wasn't," cannabis inspires questioning.

For today's meditation, sit back, relax, and question whatever you want to.

May 20

Acceptance

Acceptance is really about learning how to deal with the fact you cannot change something. You have no control. It means giving up hope, because can one fully accept something without giving up the hope for change or a different outcome? Sometimes we have to learn that things just are what they are, and nothing will ever change that specific situation. What areas of acceptance do you struggle with? Where do you have a difficult time giving up hope? Do you believe acceptance and hope can exist together side by side? Why or why not?

May 21
Faith

Faith is belief with no factual evidence, or even with contradictory factual evidence. No one can change your mind no matter how hard they try and no matter what evidence they produce. Spirituality is faith based. You have your own faith for your own reasons. What are those reasons? What brought you to have the faith you do? Have people tried to convince you otherwise? What evidence did they present to try to change your mind? Do you question your own faith? Examine and observe your relationship with faith.

May 22
Desire

Desire, an intense longing for something. What is it you desire? What do you crave in your life? Some desires are enhanced by the use of cannabis, and not just sexual ones. Cannabis does allow you to lower walls and inhibitions easily, allowing you to explore your desires. Meditate on your desires and what you would like to delve into more fully.

May 23
Be honest with yourself

Cannabis reveals much to you about yourself, often with quick, stabbing, deep revelations. It just hits you, and sometimes this smack in the face will leave you reeling. Because cannabis has this effect on the psyche, almost like a key unlocking a hidden door to allow revelations to come to light, it encourages the user to be extremely honest with him- or herself. It's difficult to lie to yourself when you are high. The truth comes crashing through your walls and says, "Stop! That isn't right!" When you lie to yourself when you aren't high and then light up? Oh yeah, weed is going to call you out on what you are doing. Be honest with yourself. Today let the weed fish around in your brain a bit. What haven't you been completely honest about? Admit to yourself what you need to and move on from there.

May 24

Breathe it in: lilac oil

Lilac corresponds with beauty, love, purification, and revealing past lives.

Decide your purpose for working with the oil. Choose what correspondence(s) you want to focus on for this session. Lilac is a beautiful, rich floral scent highly associated with the joys brought with true love. You may want to use this oil with the intent to draw your true love to you, or to celebrate the love you already have. This can be used to celebrate any love—including love for yourself. Lilac is also said to reveal your past lives to you—a peak experience accompanied by the scent of this oil can help you see into your soul's history.

Prepare your meditation area ahead of time. You may want to use a diffuser to which you can add a few drops of oil. Use a self-lighting charcoal tablet in a fireproof container, and once the tablet is lit, add a few drops of oil to it for an intense burst of the scent. If you want to use the oil on your skin, be sure to add it to a carrier oil first. To keep it simple, sniff the oil from the bottle.

Use the oil in your chosen method. Close your eyes and inhale the scent deeply and slowly several times before allowing yourself to breathe normally again. Immerse yourself in the scent so that you feel its aura all around you. If you need to, take more slow, deep breaths to increase the intensity of the scent.

What feelings does this scent invoke in you? Does it bring back memories? Do you have a connection to this scent?

Feel free to add music to this meditation.

May 25

Inner guidance

Seeking guidance when faced with a decision is a pretty common thing to do. We may reach out to our family, friends, professionals, or people we know who have had to make a similar decision. We ask for help when we are lost or searching for something we cannot find. Some people turn to their deities in prayer for guidance.

Another way to receive guidance is to ask our subconscious for it. We don't have to have a major decision to make. We don't have to be lost or searching for something. We can just check in with our higher self to ask for guidance in our daily life.

Check in with your higher self. What message of guidance do you have waiting for you today?

May 26
Inspirational inklings

"Like the sea, I am calm and indifferent. Like the wind, I have no particular direction."

—Lao Tzu[10]

Music with ocean sounds would be an ideal accompaniment for this meditation. Imagine yourself floating on the waves of the sea, bobbing from crest to crest, letting the wind steer your way. Allow the image in your mind to float effortlessly, still, carried away on the waves. Feel yourself moving with the water, never against it.

How do you become calm?

May 27
Chant

"The sun grows strong,
the nights less long.
With the moisture of the dew,
life begins anew."

This chant is perfect to do in the morning, while the dew is still on the grass and plants, especially if you have a

---

10. Lao Tzu, *The Tao Te Ching of Lao Tzu*, trans. Brian Browne Walker (St. Martin's Press, 1995), 20.

place in which to do it outside. It is refreshing and promises of goodness to come.

Repeat this chant throughout your meditation.

Try saying it in different intonations and at different speeds until you find your match.

How does this chant make you feel?

May 28

Trance dance

The calendar year is hitting the halfway point. Look back over changes you have encountered since the beginning of the year. How about the changes that have occurred since this time last year? Life is about change; it is the greatest constant.

Change is how we grow, how we learn, how we adapt.

Choose a song that helps you celebrate change.

I love "The Humming" from Enya for this change-embracing trance dance meditation.

When you are ready, begin moving with the music. Block out everything but the sound of the music.

If physical limitations require it, remain seated while moving to the music.

You can "dance" with whatever body parts you want to use. Feel free to move in whatever way feels the most pleasing to you.

Allow the music to wash over and consume you.

Where does it take you?

May 29

Got the munchies: apricots

Prepare a bowl of apricots by removing the pits.

After dosing, get into your comfy spot and set the apricots right by you. This meditation is going to focus on your taste buds and other sensations. Keep your eyes closed so that you are not relying on your sense of sight. Use your sense of smell to take in the scent of the apricots. Pay extreme attention to what you are doing as you take a bite. Feel your teeth sink into the apricot. Experience the textures and flavor, singling them out as much as possible. Take your time and enjoy the apricot. Use this type of meditation anytime you are eating for a fuller, richer connection with your food.

May 30

Inner witness

Your subconscious knows everything you have done; it is your inner witness. It follows you around like a camera crew, filming and documenting everything. Your subconscious remembers everything about you that you have forgotten. It keeps everything stored and locked away for a time when it might be needed—whether it ever is or not. All information is filed and stored where the subconscious directs it to go. When it needs to recall information, it pulls it out and then attempts to get your attention, which can be very difficult to do if you are not in tune with your subconscious. Call it a nagging thought, sudden revelation, or the little voice inside your head—these are all ways of the subconscious trying to break through to get its message across.

Today, connect with your subconscious. Check in to see what messages you have been missing.

May 31
Breathwork

By now, spring is in full bloom. The drudge of winter has been exfoliated off, and life feels good and new again. As you breathe in, think to yourself a positive word to reflect how you feel. Don't think hard. Just whatever enters your mind first. Perhaps you are happy, elated, relieved. Maybe you didn't have that great of a day though. That's okay. On your exhale, think of a word you need to rid yourself of: "stress," "tiredness," "apathy." Alternate back and forth with your breaths. Bring the positive in, let the negative out. Continue until you can no longer easily think of words to use.

✳ JUNE SHOPPING LIST ✳

Alexandrite (June 14)

Dried lavender buds (June 22)

Berries (at least three different types) (June 24)

Lavender essential oil (June 26)

June 1
Growing together

As summer approaches, now is the time where we reach out and grow, just as the natural world around us does. We are at the point in the cycle of the year where we flower and begin to bear fruit. Our ideas and plans should be coming to fruition. When we grow and rest in sync with the natural world, we live our lives with the same rhythm of the universe. We follow the ebb and flow of life cycles. Evaluate where you are with your goals and plans. Have you lost sight of your path? Do you need to put supports in place to help increase your growth? Is everything right on track and in sync with how it should be?

June 2
Wanderlust

As schools begin letting out for the summer, many people take off for vacations. Whether you have kids or not, or whether you can vacation or not, wanderlust is common this time of year. It's normal to want to get out and explore the world around you. The more alive it becomes, the more it invites you to come out and explore it in all its glory.

Let today's meditation take you on a wanderlust journey. Go wherever you want and see whatever you want to see.

June 3
Follow your heart
While it's great to get advice from other people, or to talk things out with another person, no one knows you better than your own heart does. It holds your secrets, your truths, even your lies. It knows everything about you.

In today's meditation, have a heart-to-heart with yourself. What does your heart want you to know? Where does it want to lead you?

June 4
Empowerment
You hold the keys to your own empowerment. We all do. The trick is learning how to use those keys and knowing which key goes to which lock. Other people may attempt to hold you back, throw up more locks, or to smother your efforts. You do not have to let them. The choice is yours. Find the key to unlock your voice. Who tries to

stifle your voice? Who doesn't want to hear what you have to say? Unlock your voice in your meditation, encourage yourself to use it and claim it as a part of your own empowerment.

June 5
Chill lounge

Catching fireflies as a child has always been one of my most favorite, most vivid childhood memories. Being outside after dark was a big deal. Running around in the dark over five acres of land to play with the fireflies or lightning bugs (we called them both) was when I felt most free. If there was a full moon to light my way, that was even better.

Remember back to a moment as a child—running, playing, not a care in the world. Find your happiest moment and a song that refreshes these feelings for you.

My favorite is "A Spark in the Night" by Gary Stadler and Singh Kaur.

Play your music while you are in your comfy spot. Let not only the music but any lyrics flow over you, and listen deeply and intently. Where does the music take you? How does it make you feel?

June 6
Elevate

Rise above the day-to-day hassles and negativities in today's meditation. In the grand scheme of life, these things mean nothing. Rise above them and put them behind you. You do not need to participate in things that bring you down. While it can be almost impossible to avoid negativity when there is so much of it, you can always use a cleansing, elevating meditation to rise above it so the negativity cannot touch you. Visualize yourself above the negativity, floating at peace. Allow a wave of positivity to wash over the negativity, cleansing and washing away the garbage below you. Come back down to a freshly cleansed ground, free of negativities, when you are ready.

June 7
Born in the clouds

Today's meditation should be done outside or near a window. You can do this meditation whether or not there are clouds in the sky. If there are clouds, begin by focusing on them before you close your eyes. If there aren't any, visualize big fluffy white clouds in the sky. Let them assume the shapes they want to. What shapes are born in the clouds? What message do the clouds hold for you?

June 8
Nature's way
Nature's way is to follow the cycle of the year. Rest is followed by rebirth, growth, decline, and then death—the period of rest. The cycle repeats over and over, never changing. When we follow along with the flow of the natural world, we literally feel better. Working with these energies instead of against them is beneficial. Now is the season of growth. Evaluate how well you live your life in accordance with the cycle of life. Are your plans coming to fruition? If needed, what adjustments can you make to get your life back in sync with the energies around you?

June 9
Embrace life's pleasures
Life brings both pleasure and pain. It is because of the unavoidable pains we will all suffer that we need to make sure we take the time to appreciate and embrace all of the pleasures life has to offer. Spend today's meditation embracing and appreciating the pleasures you have in your life.

June 10

Call of the wild: birdsong

Do an online search for "bird song."

Find a bird song that is a good length for your meditation time or use a repeat feature.

Play the song and meditate on it as you listen.

Do you like this sound? Dislike the sound?

Let the sound encompass you.

How does it make you feel?

June 11

Inspirational inklings

"Children are inherently mindful, but as we get older it's a quality that many of us lose. We spend much of our time drifting through our days on automatic pilot, thinking about the past or daydreaming about the future."

—Anna Black[11]

Black opens her chapter "What Is Mindfulness?" with this statement. I don't know about you, but I can guarantee I have been guilty of dwelling in the past and daydreaming about the future many hundreds of thousands of times. Spend your meditation today completely in the

11. Anna Black, *A Year of Living Mindfully: Week-by-Week Mindfulness Meditations for a More Contented and Fulfilled Life* (New York: Cico Books, 2015), 9.

now. Notice each moment, listen, use your sense of scent; what do you feel? Focus on simply being in the now and escort out any other thoughts which pop up. Be mindful of your present.

June 12
Respect

Respect has made an interesting journey. Once, it was given away freely to everyone, especially to people you didn't know or to people who were your elders. As a society, this isn't true anymore. Now we demand respect be earned. It's too early to tell how this shift is going to pan out for future generations.

No matter what society says, you yourself choose who you are going to respect, and the first place you need to look is at yourself. Do you hold yourself in high regard? Do you have good self-esteem? Sadly, many people do not, so if you don't, you are not alone. Use your meditation time today to remind yourself: You deserve respect. Not only from others, but from yourself. Until you have respect for yourself, it's very difficult to obtain it from anyone else. Today, try repeating this mantra: "I respect myself." The more you say it, the more you will begin to feel it. Allow this short mantra to empower you and give yourself the respect you deserve.

June 13

Be fearless

Fear, anxiety, uncertainty—all these things hold us back. While some fears are justified (fear of fire, for example), we often have everyday fears we don't particularly notice. Very common is a fear of failure or embarrassment, which can keep us from doing or saying the things that are very much in our hearts or minds.

Today, be fearless in your meditation. Say the things you would like to say but feel you can't. Put those hidden fears out into the universe. Let the universe give you the strength to say what you need to. Practice being fearless. Like anything, with practice you get better at doing something. Practicing being fearless will help you become fearless.

June 14

Get stoned: alexandrite

Alexandrite is a blue-green stone that resonates with good luck, good self-esteem, and centering oneself.

Choose one or more of these qualities that calls to you. Charging a stone emphasizing all three traits makes it an ideal stone to use in situations such as legal issues or job interviews.

Get into your comfy spot and hold the stone in your hand out in front of you.

Examine the stone with your eyes and your fingers.

Feel the stone as you hold it tightly in your hand.
Hold the stone close to your heart.
Meditate on the stone and how it feels to you.
Carry this stone with you whenever you feel the need.

June 15

Busy as a bee

Our society is constantly on the go or in search of constant stimulation. Like bees, we buzz from flower to flower in a tizzy, constantly looking for more. There is one huge difference, however. For a bee, their life depends on staying busy. Does yours? Probably not. In fact, your life would probably be a lot less hectic if you toned down your bee-like activities. Meditate today on the unnecessary buzzing activities you have. How can you simplify your life so you do not have to be busy as a bee?

June 16

The Green Man

If you can, do this meditation outside. Meditations dealing with nature are more effective when you are able to perform them in nature.

The Green Man is a representation of the cycle of life. He represents rebirth and growth. In the summer months, the Green Man is depicted with full, lush green foliage. He watches over the natural world, protecting those under his care.

Today, visualize living out in the woods and being under the Green Man's care. Allow your imagination to create the world it wants to and let it lead to an encounter with the Green Man. What is your encounter like? What message does the Green Man have for you?

June 17
The spirit of trees

This meditation should be done outdoors in a location where trees are present, and you can sit on the ground (or in a chair) with your back up against one. Trees have a calming, grounding effect to them. Feel the connection with the tree. Just sit there and feel the tree against your back. Feel free to put your hands behind you and feel the bark too. Is it smooth? Rough? The spirit of the tree has a message for you. Spend time communing with the tree and let the message come to you.

June 18
Chant

"In this time,
in this place,
I create around me,
sacred space."

This is the perfect chant to put yourself into the ideal frame of mind for a spiritual encounter with deity or other form of spirit. Create around you a safe, sacred aura in which to connect with the universe.

Repeat this chant throughout your meditation.

Try saying it in different intonations and at different speeds until you find your match.

How does this chant make you feel?

What does it mean to you?

June 19

Grace

Grace is a subjective concept that can mean different things to different people. For some it is the ability to remain calm and objective in difficult situations or crises. For others, it is the elegance of exceptional manners. Others, still, see grace as the ability to physically move effortlessly in an ethereal manner. Meditate on what grace means to you. How can you incorporate more grace into your own life?

June 20

A midsummer night's dream

If possible, this meditation should be done outside at night, preferably in a wooded area.

If mystical creatures we cannot see do exist, they will be filled with merriment tonight. Fairies are said to be highly active on midsummer's nights. Tonight, in your meditation, visit with the Fae. Who do you meet? What do they look like? It is said if you eat or drink anything while in the presence of fairies, you will be trapped in their world. You may want to play it safe and keep your activities centered on dancing and games instead. Celebrate with the fairies and say goodbye when you part ways.

June 21

Make a seasonal offering

Start the new season off with an offering. Choose an emotional, active, or physical offering. (Or all three!) Give your offering to your deities, your higher power, or the universe at large.

An emotional offering can be "Love, kindness, and good health to all." It can be a special prayer.

Active offerings include things like providing lawn care to an elderly person, volunteering at a day camp or soup kitchen, or helping to maintain a community garden.

You may choose a physical offering such as "firsts" harvested from your own garden, or other foods you prepare yourself.

Meditate on what offerings you can give.

June 22

Smoke the herb: lavender

Lavender is an incredible herb to add in with cannabis. It produces an even more relaxed effect, and the scent is intoxicating. Lavender corresponds to happiness, healing, love, peace, and sleep.

Combine your cannabis with some dried lavender buds. Use a mix of about 70 percent cannabis to 30 percent lavender, but you can adjust that according to your preferences.

When combining herbs with cannabis for the first time, always resort back to "slow and low." You are introducing a new combination of acids, proteins, and terpenes to your system. Give yourself time to see how it affects you, and that's all you have to do. Meditate on your reactions: How does it make you feel? Do you like it? How can you use this combination further in your practices?

June 23

Express your individuality

One of the great benefits of cannabis is the effect it has on opening and broadening your creativity. Use that creativity today to express your individuality in your meditation. If there were no limits (and in your meditations there aren't!), what would you change about your appearance to express your individuality? You can give yourself a lion's mane or a unicorn's horn or superpowers, whatever describes you the best. Use your creativity to design your most unique expression of you.

June 24
Got the munchies: berries

After dosing, get into your comfy spot and set the berries right by you. This meditation is going to focus on your taste buds and other sensations. Keep your eyes closed so that you are not relying on your sense of sight. Use your sense of smell to take in the scent of each berry before you eat it. Can you identify it from the scent? Pay extreme attention to what you are doing as you take a bite. Feel your teeth sink into the berry. Experience the textures and flavor, singling them out as much as possible. Take your time and enjoy each of the berries, testing yourself to see if you can identify each one by the taste and scent. Use this type of meditation anytime you are eating for a fuller, richer connection with your food.

June 25
Wanderlust

Let your mind take you on a vacation today.

Where would you like to go? What do you want to see and do? You don't need tickets or baggage or security lines, just let your mind go to where you would like to be.

Spend as much time there as you want. You may hop to different locations or focus on one. This is your mental vacation, so take it however and wherever you want. Let yourself relax, smile, and enjoy.

June 26
Breathe it in: lavender oil

Lavender oil corresponds with healing, peace, sleep, love, and happiness. It is very relaxing and incredible for helping you to fall asleep.

Decide your purpose for working with the oil. Choose what correspondence(s) you want to focus on for this session. Do you need some peace and healing in your life? Having difficulties sleeping? Or perhaps you just want to focus on love and happiness?

Prepare your meditation area ahead of time. You may want to use a diffuser to which you can add a few drops of oil. Use a self-lighting charcoal tablet in a fireproof container, and once the tablet is lit, add a few drops of oil to it for an intense burst of the scent. If you want to use the oil on your skin, be sure to add it to a carrier oil first. To keep it simple, sniff the oil from the bottle.

Use the oil in your chosen method. Close your eyes and inhale the scent deeply and slowly several times before allowing yourself to breathe normally again. Immerse yourself in the scent so that you feel its aura all around you. If you need to, take more slow, deep breaths to increase the intensity of the scent.

What feelings does this scent invoke in you? Does it bring back memories? Do you have a connection to this scent?

Feel free to add music to this meditation.

June 27

Magic in the making

If you can, do this meditation outside under the night sky.

We live on a giant rock with a diameter of just over 7,900 miles that travels around a giant ball of gas and has existed for billions of years. You are an exceptional being made up of 37.2 trillion cells. You are quite literally made of stardust. What could be more magical than all of that? Use today's meditation to visit the birth of the universe. Visualize as stars turn supernova, exploding into stardust that reassembles into new life. Experience the true magic of your existence.

June 28

Inspirational inklings

"Picture yourself in any position that you like. Standing, sitting, lying down, whatever is easiest for you to imagine.

Now look at that mental picture of yourself. What you see, in this exercise, is a you who is always looking away from yourself. Always looking outside of yourself. You are facing the wrong way!"

—Wayne W. Dyer[12]

Did you see the back side of yourself when you first envisioned yourself as Dyer described? Were you surprised at his words that you were looking the wrong way? Spend time today in your meditation envisioning yourself from the front. Look upon your own face, into your own eyes.

June 29
Trance dance

Summer is the time for surf and sand, even if you don't live anywhere near it. Celebrate the vitality of life with an energetic trance dance that brings to you the waves crashing on the beach, splashing in the foam. Dress the part if you want by throwing on your swimsuit. Enjoy and have fun with this carefree dance.

I like "The Beachside of Life" by Sunlounger.

When you are ready, begin moving with the music. Block out everything but the sound of the music.

---

12. Wayne W. Dyer, *Your Sacred Self: Making the Decision to Be Free* (New York: HarperCollins Publishers, 1995), 5.

If physical limitations require it, remain seated while moving to the music.

You can "dance" with whatever body parts you want to use. Feel free to move in whatever way feels the most pleasing to you.

Allow the music to wash over and consume you.

Where does it take you?

June 30

Breathwork

Take some deep meditative breaths as you reflect back over your month.

Focus on anything new you learned, new knowledge you obtained.

As you breathe deeply, in and out, slowly, visualize this new information integrating into your spirit, your mind, your body, wherever this new information will do the most good. Where is it needed? Direct it there.

"File" all your learnings while breathing deeply and slowly. Pace yourself. Give yourself time to relive moments as much as desired.

A few examples:

New information: "I learned a new recipe this month and I really enjoyed it."

This information can be sent several places. Send it to your taste buds so they remember how much they enjoyed it! Reflect on the taste so that in your mind you can taste it again. Send this information to your heart. This recipe made you feel good. Send this information to your brain. Store this recipe for future use so you can use it again.

New information: "I learned to connect with my higher self."

This information can be sent to your heart because it makes you feel good. Send it to your brain so you can repeat the performance in the future. But also send this to your spirit because that is where this happens and is felt the most.

✳ JULY SHOPPING LIST ✳

Ruby (July 13)

Dried crushed damiana (July 16)

Melon chunks (at least 3 different types) (July 25)

Lemongrass essential oil (July 29)

July 1
Spiritual sustenance

Your body needs nourishment. Your mind needs nourishment. Your spirituality also needs nourishment. Meditation is but one form of spiritual sustenance. How else do you feed your spirituality? Evaluate your spiritual diet. Are you getting all the nutrients you need? Do you partake in a bit of variety to keep your spiritual life energized and fresh?

July 2
Body work

In today's meditation, check in with your body. Get into your comfy spot, and then give your body a good thorough once over. How is everything feeling and working? Work from the tips of your toes to the top of your head, checking each inch as you go. Send it love and a healing, cleansing white light. When you are done, give yourself a hug.

July 3
Manifest your desires

As the year progresses, you should be working on those goals you wanted accomplished, the desires you want manifested into your life. Today, meditate on where you are with those goals. Are some complete? Are some stagnant? Have your goals changed? Have you added in new or tossed out old ones? What is your next move to manifest your desires?

July 4
Freedom

Today is a great day to celebrate freedom. In your meditation, think about what freedom means to you. We have many different kinds of freedoms, but we are also still restrained in many ways. In what ways do you celebrate your freedom? What freedoms do you want but find they are out of reach?

July 5
Child's play

Summer is a time for fun and games and forgetting how old we are. It's a time to go outside and play under the sun and feel young again. Meditate on how you liked to play as a child. What games and outdoor fun did you have in the summer? Think back to how you felt and what life was like for you then. How can you incorporate child's play back into your life?

July 6

Nature therapy

This meditation should be performed outside, either day or night, in a nice, quiet location where you can lie down on the ground. You may want a pillow for comfort.

There is no better way to ground yourself than by literally lying down on the ground. Connect as much of your body as you can with the earth. Spread out your arms and legs in a comfortable position and allow yourself to sink to the ground. Relax yourself fully. Visualize healing energies coming toward you from all living things around you—trees, flowers, the very grass you are lying on. All of it sends healing energy to you. Allow the healing energy to absorb into you and do whatever it needs to. Let it refresh your body and mend any issues it finds along the way.

July 7

Liberation

Liberation is defined as the act of setting someone free from imprisonment, slavery, or oppression. It is not always others, however, that keep us held in one of these circumstances. We do it to ourselves. We imprison ourselves in a life that doesn't truly work for us. While not actual slavery, we call ourselves "slaves to the job" to hopefully be able to provide for ourselves and to play keep up with the Joneses in the never-ending quest for the next great new electronic gadget. We oppress ourselves by not doing and saying the things we really want.

Today, let the cannabis lower your walls to focus on these areas. How do you imprison yourself? What are you a slave to? What would true liberation look like? What liberating steps can you take in your life?

July 8
Perception

Your point of view drastically affects how you perceive things. It's also often extremely difficult to see things from someone else's point of view because you can never fully put yourself into their shoes. Your perception is affected by all the events that have happened in your life. Every moment you have lived in the past affects how you see things in the present and in the future. Events may happen to you that cause you to adjust your point of view, which may in turn change how you perceive things. This is part of what makes us unique individual beings. None of us have had the exact same experiences, so each of us has a different and unique point of view.

Today, meditate on a time when you did not see eye to eye with someone else. Now that time has passed, and your point of view has changed in other ways, do you still see the situation the same way you did then? Using what you know about that person, imagine how the situation might look through their eyes. Are you able to more clearly see their point of view even if you do not agree with it?

July 9

Trust your dreams

There are two different types of dreams: those when you go to sleep at night and those you fantasize over during the day. It may be your dream job, dream date, dream home, dream vacation. It's a dream—a reality you don't expect to come about. There within lies the problem: we simply do not expect our dreams to come true. Without expectation, they will not become reality. Change your expectations for your dreams, and you can begin working on moving them from the fantasy realm to the real world. Meditate today on a small dream. One that isn't impossible (you aren't going to turn into a unicorn) but is probable—such as a vacation or other smaller dream. What is keeping you from making this dream a reality? What steps can you take to move it from fantasy to reality?

July 10
Call of the wild: windchimes

Do an online search for "windchimes sounds."

Find a windchimes clip that is a good length for your meditation time or use a repeat feature.

Play the song and meditate on it as you listen.

Do you like this sound? Dislike the sound?

Let the sound encompass you.

How does it make you feel?

July 11
Energy healing

Do this meditation during the day under the rays of the sun (not in the shade). If you burn easily, be sure to use sunscreen, a hat, and other protection.

Summer is a time for getting into shape and working on your physical body. Being outside provides fresh air and sunlight, and these two together can be very healing and a great energy booster. Find a comfortable position either on the ground or in a chair and close your eyes. Feel the rays of the sun as they shine down on you, spreading their warmth. Visualize those rays as the sun's energy healing your body, mind, and soul, energizing it. Let the sun's rays recharge you.

July 12

Growth

Vegetation is at its height of growth for the season. First harvests are coming in, and plants are fertile and producing the fruits of their biological labors. Today, be a plant. Imagine your roots have grown deep into the ground. They are well nourished, well watered. Your stalk or stem is strong yet pliable. You can stand tall yet bend easily with the wind. Your foliage is lush and richly green. You are in full bloom. Do you produce a fruit? Vegetable? Nuts? Seeds? Whatever you are, see yourself as fertile and abundantly full.

July 13

Get stoned: ruby

Ruby is a red stone that resonates with vitality, power, courage, integrity, joy, and prosperity, and it prevents nightmares.

Choose one or more of these qualities that calls to you. Think of different combinations you could combine together. Do you have nightmares? With the added power and courage, it is the perfect stone to sleep with in your pillowcase. Are you a hard worker that refuses to sell out? More power, courage, integrity, joy, and prosperity to you for sticking to your beliefs.

Create a stone that works for you.

Get into your comfy spot and hold the stone in your hand out in front of you.

Examine the stone with your eyes and your fingers.

Feel the stone as you hold it tightly in your hand.

Hold the stone close to your heart.

Meditate on the stone and how it feels to you.

Carry this stone with you whenever you feel the need.

July 14
Inspirational inklings
"Your body is not your self; you are much more than this body. You are life without boundaries."

—Thich Nhat Hanh[13]

A peak experience helps you to experience the feeling of being a life without boundaries. Meditate today on how you can apply this feeling, this knowledge that you are indeed life without boundaries, to your everyday life.

July 15
Reconnect with nature
What is your earliest memory of an experience out in nature? Did you enjoy it? Hate it? What were you doing? Recall the memory in as much detail as you can and

---

13. Thich Nhat Hanh, *The Art of Living: Peace and Freedom in the Here and Now* (New York: HarperOne, 2017), 52.

remember how you felt about it. Would you feel the same way in a similar situation today?

July 16
Smoke the herb: damiana

Damiana is an aphrodisiac and is also used for attracting love.

Combine your cannabis with some dried ground damiana. Use a mix of about 80 percent cannabis to 20 percent damiana, but you can adjust that according to your preferences.

When combining herbs with cannabis for the first time, always resort back to "slow and low." You are introducing a new combination of acids, proteins, and terpenes to your system. Give yourself time to see how it affects you, and that's all you have to do. Meditate on your reactions: How does it make you feel? Do you like it? How can you use this combination further in your practices?

July 17
Chill lounge

The heat of summer is upon us. Plants flourish as the first harvests begin to ripen. The strength of the sun is at its height as his rays shine down upon the earth, nourishing her inhabitants. It is a time to celebrate the sun, the toil, the sweat, the growth, the power. It is a time to celebrate the gods, or other masculine aspects.

Choose a song that reflects the masculine aspect of the summer to you.

I use "Cernunnos" by Omnia.

Play your music while you are in your comfy spot. Let not only the music but any lyrics flow over you, and listen deeply and intently. Where does the music take you? How does it make you feel?

July 18
Confidence

Confidence is defined as the belief you can rely on something or someone. Do you have confidence in yourself? Can you rely on yourself to keep you safe? To allow yourself to grow? To make the right choices? Today, evaluate your level of confidence in yourself. Do you trust yourself in some areas but not so much in others? What can you do to increase confidence in yourself?

July 19
Instinct

Chickens are a very instinctual animal. They hatch from their eggs and, whether there is a mother hen around or not, they are able to get up within minutes, start walking, and begin feeding themselves. They do not have to be taught any of this. It just happens. They automatically know what to do.

Your instincts may not be that fine-tuned, but you can learn how to rely on them simply by using them more often. Practicing using your instincts builds your confidence and strengthens your connection. Let today's meditation focus on your instincts. What do they want you to know for the present?

July 20
Sensuality
Sensuality is a word that often gets a bad rap. While it can pertain to lewdness, the main definition is that sensuality pertains to the indulgence and gratification of the senses. Since cannabis heightens the senses, sensuality and cannabis go hand in hand. Spend today's meditation focusing on each of the different senses and their relationship to cannabis. Focus on its taste, its scent, the sound when it burns, and how it makes you feel.

July 21
Volatility
During long hot summers, tempers flare more easily. Crime rates go up. Wildfires spread due to the dryness of plants and the land. Summer, in some places, becomes

quite volatile. Today, no matter where you are, spend your meditation sending cooling, calming thoughts to those around you and to the universe. Send your positive chilled vibrations to where they are needed most.

July 22
Reflection

Take some time today to reflect on how things are going for you so far this year. How are you doing on your goals? Evaluate where you are at and compare to your expectations. You don't need to judge or chastise yourself if you aren't where you expected. Simply acknowledge where you are now and reflect on what you have accomplished so far.

July 23
Be bold

Ever have one of those moments when you wish you had said or done something but didn't because you were scared of what others would think? You knew you should stand up but just couldn't find the strength to do it?

Replay the episode in your meditation today. But this time, allow yourself to stand up and be bold. Say what you need to say. It won't change the past, but it will allow you to get off your chest what you need to.

July 24
Getting to know yourself

Cannabis is well known for the way it allows you to see yourself from an outsider's perspective. You are able to step out of your actions and beliefs and truly see yourself with an objective eye. This can reveal both wonderful and scary things about yourself. Learning the truth, whether good or bad, is a positive aspect. The truth, when unpleasant, allows us to make changes for the better.

Today, get to know yourself better. Allow the walls to drop and take an objective view. Ask the universe to show you a not-so-great moment. Can you see the event more objectively now? What can you learn from this experience?

July 25
Got the munchies: melon

After dosing, get into your comfy spot and set a bowl of melon chunks right by you. Have three different varieties. This meditation is going to focus on your taste buds and other sensations. Keep your eyes closed so that you are not relying on your sense of sight. Use your sense of smell to take in the scent of each melon chunk before you eat it. Can you identify it from the scent? Pay extreme attention to what you are doing as you take a bite. Feel your teeth sink into the melon. Experience the textures and flavor, singling them out as much as possible. Take your time and enjoy each of the chunks, testing yourself to see if you can identify each one by the taste and scent. Use this type of meditation anytime you are eating for a fuller, richer connection with your food.

July 26
Inspirational inklings

"Stillness—emptiness or *shunyata* in Buddhist teaching— is synonymous with peace. Awareness in the presence of stillness walks hand in hand with love."

—Stephan Gray[14]

We often find ourselves uncomfortable in times of silence because we have been taught stillness is negative. Our society emphasizes activity and always being on the go. Being on the go leaves you drained. Stillness and peace allow you to refresh and revitalize. What beliefs do you have about stillness? Adjust your perceptions, if necessary, to see how stillness, peace, and love are all intertwined.

14. Stephen Gray, ed. *Cannabis and Spirituality: An Explorer's Guide to an Ancient Plant Spirit Ally* (Rochester, VT: Park Street Press, 2017), 5.

July 27
Chant

"Like the rays from the sun,
I am strong.
Like the beams from the moon,
I am pure."

Whether at dawn, daylight, twilight, or night, this chant connects you to the dichotomy of the relationship of the sun and moon. We can, and should, connect with aspects of both these celestial bodies. Envision the rays from the sun entering you as you chant about them. Alternate by envisioning the beams from the moon entering you as you chant about them. Feel yourself growing stronger and purer.

Repeat this chant throughout your meditation.

Try saying it in different intonations and at different speeds until you find your match.

How does this chant make you feel?

What does it mean to you?

July 28
Wonderland

When Alice went down the rabbit hole, she entered Wonderland, a strange and different world where the impossible was possible.

Today, let your imagination take you down a rabbit hole into your own creation of Wonderland. What does it look like? Who do you meet? What adventure will you encounter?

July 29

Breathe it in: lemongrass oil

Lemongrass oil is cleansing, and it purifies. It gives an energy boost and increases psychic awareness.

Decide your purpose for working with the oil. Choose what correspondence(s) you want to focus on for this session. Lemongrass is a great scent to work with for cleansing, so you can always use it in a meditation for cleansing your aura, chakras, or both. Intuition is also highly enhanced with the use of cannabis, so combining lemongrass oil for a boost in psychic awareness is perfect for any type of divination, intuitive, or self-exploration workings.

Prepare your meditation area ahead of time. You may want to use a diffuser to which you can add a few drops of oil. Use a self-lighting charcoal tablet in a fireproof container, and once the tablet is lit, add a few drops of oil to it for an intense burst of the scent. If you want to use the oil on your skin, be sure to add it to a carrier oil first. To keep it simple, sniff the oil from the bottle.

Use the oil in your chosen method. Close your eyes and inhale the scent deeply and slowly several times before allowing yourself to breathe normally again. Immerse yourself in the scent so that you feel its aura all around you. If you need to, take more slow, deep breaths to increase the intensity of the scent.

What feelings does this scent invoke in you? Does it bring back memories? Do you have a connection to this scent?

Feel free to add music to this meditation.

July 30

Trance dance

In the deep heart of summer, I like to do this trance dance meditation outside after dark. I want to feel my own primal instincts join in with the natural world around me, so in my backyard is key for me. Imagine connecting with your native ancestors dancing around a bonfire as early peoples the world over did. Feel your biological connection with earth. If you cannot find a place outside to do this meditation, perform it near an open window.

Find a song that invokes a primal connection with nature in you.

My favorite is "Gratitude Joy" by Anand Anugrah and Paul Avgerinos.

When you are ready, begin moving with the music. Block out everything but the sound of the music.

If physical limitations require it, remain seated while moving to the music.

You can "dance" with whatever body parts you want to use. Feel free to move in whatever way feels the most pleasing to you.

Allow the music to wash over and consume you.

Where does it take you?

July 31
Breathwork
Release some fire in your end of the month breathwork today.

Sit in a comfortable position and take in a deep breath. Hold it as long as is comfortable. As you exhale, imagine you are a fire-breathing dragon and woooooooosh your flame out. See the fire as it erupts from your lips and billows into the air.

Allow it to burn up any tensions.

Let out any feelings that are holding you down.

Release anything you have no control over.

Continue breathing your dragon breath, repeating as often as you like.

✳ AUGUST SHOPPING LIST ✳

Peridot (August 12)

Dried crushed horehound (August 13)

Patchouli essential oil (August 22)

Apple slices (at least three different varieties) (August 25)

August 1
Rhythm

This meditation is more beneficial done outside or near an open window.

Nature is filled with rhythm. From the rhythm of the tides to the rhythm of bird calls to the rhythm of your own heartbeat, nature makes its own music.

Focus on the sounds you hear. What different rhythms can you pick out?

August 2
Turn over a new leaf

In today's meditation, come up with one idea, one change you can make in your life. One new leaf you can turn over. Something small that you can change to create a new good habit or to replace a bad habit. Meditate on incorporating it into your life. When you are done with your meditation, be sure to give yourself reminders, like adding it to your phone with an alarm or writing it down on your daily calendar.

August 3
Splendor in the grass

For today's meditation, again go outside if you can. You will want to find a grassy location to lie down on. If you need a sheet or blanket for comfort, use one, but if you can tolerate lying directly on the grass, please do.

If you can't do this, then visualize lying in the grass instead.

From your view, look all around and take in the beauty of nature. Take in the big picture along with the small, right down to individual blades of grass. Hold a blade of grass in your hand as you lay back and imagine yourself the size of an ant. What would the world right around you look like from your new point of view? Spend your meditation time exploring this new world

August 4
Cycles

We live through several different cycles all at the same time. We have a daily cycle, weekly cycle, monthly cycle, yearly cycle, and seasonal cycle, just to name a few. These are natural cycles made possible by the rotation of our earth, the way it travels around the sun, and the way the moon travels around us. These are also cycles we take for granted. Today, don't take them for granted. In your meditation, focus on the rotation of the earth, the moon revolving around the earth, and then the earth revolving around the sun. Appreciate how truly amazing these cycles are.

August 5
Temptation
Temptation. We all face it. Something that we find so enticing, "no" seems an impossible answer. What temptations do you face in your life? Which ones can you pass up? Which one's can't you?

Do your temptations have something to tell you?

August 6
Clear your energy
Get in some energy maintenance today. Visualize white light coming in through the top of your head. Allow it to flow through you, veining out in every direction, covering every inch of your body. Feel the white light cleansing as it moves throughout you, leaving you feeling refreshed and renewed. When the light has done its job, visualize it leaving your body and being absorbed into the ground.

August 7
Totem animals

Whether you currently work with a totem animal or not, today, open your mind to see what animal comes to you. Go to your sacred space in your mind and wait to see who comes to visit you. The totem who shows itself to you has a message. After your meditation, use one of the many available totem animal guidebooks, or do an online search for the spiritual meaning of the animal that comes to you.

August 8
Good fortune

If you want to attract good fortune in your life, you need to focus on what good fortune would bring to you. Meditate today on what good fortune you seek, what impact it would make, and how your life would be different with it.

August 9
Gratitude

Don't save your giving of thanks for November. Learn to show and share your gratitude on a daily basis. Spend today's meditation expressing gratitude for all that you have, for all that you love, for all that is good in your life. After this meditation, make a conscious effort to take a moment to express gratitude every day in your life.

August 10
Call of the wild: forest at night
Do an online search for "forest at night."

Find a clip that is a good length for your meditation time or use a repeat feature.

Play the song and meditate on it as you listen.

Do you like this sound? Dislike the sound?

Let the sound encompass you.

How does it make you feel?

August 11
Easy does it
Take it easy today and give yourself a break. Anything crazy going on in your life? Is life hectic? Too much to do? Work getting you down? Whatever it is that is bothering you in life right now, whatever is not working out the way you want it to, just forget about it for now. Set it aside, and let your imagination take you to someplace peaceful, relaxing, and stress free.

August 12
Get stoned: peridot
Peridot is a green stone that resonates with beauty, emotional balance, health, intuition, protection, luck, and prosperity.

Choose one or more of these qualities that calls to you. Which of these qualities do you need to call into your life? How can you combine them to personalize a stone for you? Have an upcoming interview? All these qualities can apply to give you a boost. Just starting out meditating? Emotional balance and intuition are two key components of meditating—adding a peridot into your practice can help add an objective focus through emotional balance. It may also open your experience with oneness through intuition. Find what works for you.

Get into your comfy spot and hold the stone in your hand out in front of you.

Examine the stone with your eyes and your fingers.

Feel the stone as you hold it tightly in your hand.

Hold the stone close to your heart.

Meditate on the stone and how it feels to you.

Carry this stone with you whenever you feel the need.

August 13
Smoke the herb: horehound
Horehound is used for protection, increasing your mental abilities, and healing. It also dispels negativity.

Combine your cannabis with some dried ground horehound. Use a mix of about 80 percent cannabis to 20 percent horehound, but you can adjust that according to your preferences.

When combining herbs with cannabis for the first time, always resort back to "slow and low." You are introducing a new combination of acids, proteins, and terpenes to your system. Give yourself time to see how it affects you, and that's all you have to do. Meditate on your reactions: How does it make you feel? Do you like it? How can you use this combination further in your practices?

August 14
Speak up
There is a slowly disintegrating stigma in America that stereotypes people who consume cannabis. More and more that stereotype is being proven wrong as more people begin using cannabis for medical needs. The fastest way to rip that stigma from those who use cannabis is to speak out about your experience and to educate others. Meditate today on how you can be more vocal about what cannabis has done to help you. How can you educate others and help them learn the stereotypes and stigma are false?

August 15
Emotional healing
Cannabis is a great revealer, which leads to a part of its healing powers. Cannabis helps to show you what the damage is, the damage your ego hides from you to pro-

tect you from pain. Pain, however, is necessary in order to heal. Let cannabis reveal a past pain to you today. One that you have put aside and forgotten about in order to not have to deal with the pain. Today, instead of ignoring the pain, allow yourself to feel it. Grieve for whatever it is you need to. Allow the pain to flow out of you. As your heart heals, you receive blessings and love from your deities, your spirit guides, your ancestors, and the universe.

August 16
Restorative retreat
In today's meditation, visualize yourself in your own personal restorative retreat—whatever images that conjures up for you. For some it may be inside with a spa-like interior. For others, it may be a setting deep in the woods or in an open meadow. Still others may want to visualize themselves in a protective bubble floating in space, underwater, or in an entirely different manner. Whatever it is for you that allows you to put everything else aside to focus only on you.

Use your third eye to scan your body and then guide cleansing, healing energies throughout, concentrating on any areas in need.

Practice deep breathing and visualize each breath restoring you closer and closer to full energy.

Spend as much time in your meditation as you need. Do not set any time limits today.

August 17
Courage

The sun is a symbol of strength and courage. Mid-August in the US and the sun is at its full height of power (often with scorching heat). We, too, are at the full height of our power as our energy coincides with the energy of the natural world around us. This energy, this strength, helps to embolden us and to give us courage. It is in the winter we hide, but in the height of summer, we shine.

In today's meditation, think about a situation where you have been lacking courage to do what needs to be done. Draw upon the energy, the strength of the sun, to raise your own energy and strength. Meditate on what being courageous in this situation will look like. Play it out in your mind. Use your meditation as a practice run to prepare you for the real thing.

August 18
Celebrate life

This meditation should be completed outside if possible. If not, then be sure to perform it by an open window to enable a better connection with the environment.

While the sun is at his full power, life abounds. From insects to birds to mammals to plant life of all varieties, the world is alive. Take a moment to sense and appreciate the life forces all around you. Feel their energy and comprehend that they can feel your life energy as well. We often see things only from our point of view; today, for a bit, try to imagine what your energy must look like to other life forms. How would your energy feel to the grass you sit upon? The tree you sit beneath? The bird hopping across the grass? How do these life-forms see your energy? Send these other life-forms positive vibes to celebrate their life energy.

August 19
Chill lounge
Summer is slowly coming to an end. Take today to appreciate what you have accomplished so far this year. Reflect on tasks and projects completed and the journey behind them. Go ahead—pat yourself on the back. But, also let this serve as a reminder to get moving on other projects that you may be lagging on. Celebrate, yet motivate.

Choose a song that reflects the time and the theme: things are going great, just keep moving on. What song lights a spark for you?

I use "Kiva Ceremony" by Diane Arkenstone.

Play your music while you are in your comfy spot. Let not only the music but any lyrics flow over you, and listen deeply and intently. Where does the music take you? How does it make you feel?

August 20
Bountiful harvest

While families and farmers are gathering the fruits of their gardens and crops, it is now time to begin gathering the harvests of the crops you have planted. The energy is still strong, but the signs point the way to the rest time of winter that is soon to come. It is time for your goals to be coming to fruition. Gather in the crops of your goal completions. Put more energy toward goals that need more tender, loving care in order to thrive. Pick ripe goals and store their experience.

August 21
Radiant light

Take a moment to go outside and soak up some radiant light. Close your eyes, turn your face to the sky, and let the sun shine down on it. Even if it is overcast—you know the sun is there, just blocked from view. Its light is still there shining down on you. Feel the radiant light on the skin on your face, your skin. Feel the warmth of the radiant light as it passes through your skin and into your being. Your soul. You are a part of the radiant light of the sun.

August 22
Breathe it in: patchouli oil
Patchouli is known for its aphrodisiac properties, but it is also used for protection and divination.

Decide your purpose for working with the oil. Choose what correspondence(s) you want to focus on for this session. If you don't have a reason to use patchouli for its aphrodisiac properties—no worries! But if you do have a reason, there is no sense in passing the opportunity up if available.

Patchouli is also wonderful for protection and divination, which means you can use patchouli in a free-thought prophetic meditation. Do this by allowing the universe to take you where it will and show you what it wants. It will be your job to read and decipher what you see.

Prepare your meditation area ahead of time. You may want to use a diffuser to which you can add a few drops of oil. Use a self-lighting charcoal tablet in a fireproof container, and once the tablet is lit, add a few drops of oil to it for an intense burst of the scent. If you want to use the oil on your skin, be sure to add it to a carrier oil first. To keep it simple, sniff the oil from the bottle.

Use the oil in your chosen method. Close your eyes and inhale the scent deeply and slowly several times before allowing yourself to breathe normally again. Immerse yourself in the scent so that you feel its aura all around you. If you need to, take more slow, deep breaths to increase the intensity of the scent.

What feelings does this scent invoke in you? Does it bring back memories? Do you have a connection to this scent?

Feel free to add music to this meditation.

August 23
Inspirational inklings
"Sometimes, running away means you're headed in the exact right direction."

—Alice Hoffman[15]

Have you ever found yourself in a situation like this? Turning away from something is not always a bad thing! It can put us on the track we are meant to be on. Have you missed necessary turns by running toward something when you should have gone another direction? Reflect on how your choices have led you to where you are now.

---

15. Alice Hoffman, *Practical Magic* (New York: Penguin, 2003), n.p.

August 24
Spiritual truth

Spirituality is the concept of being more concerned with your soul or spirit than you are with material possessions. It is also a circular pattern.

When you are more concerned with your soul than you are with material possessions, you simply do not need or want more material possessions. This frees up resources such as time and money to put toward soul-enriching experiences instead. The more enriched your soul, the fewer material possessions craved.

Meditate on this cycle. What soul-enriching experiences would you like to have? Follow your truth to find your way to them.

August 25
Got the munchies: apples

After dosing, get into your comfy spot and set a bowl of apple slices next to you. You are using three different types of apples. This meditation is going to focus on your taste buds and other sensations. Keep your eyes closed so that you are not relying on your sense of sight. Use your sense of smell to take in the scent of each slice before you eat it. Can you identify the variety from the scent? Pay extreme attention to what you are doing as you take a bite. Feel your teeth sink into the apple. Experience the textures and flavor, singling them out as much as possible. Take your time and enjoy each of the slices, testing yourself to see if you can identify each one by the taste and scent. Use this type of meditation anytime you are eating for a fuller, richer connection with your food.

August 26
Higher knowledge
Let's face it. Cannabis can help bring out the stupid in people, but it can also bring out incredible insightfulness. Partakers all remember their first "deep thoughts" moment, though chances are, they don't remember what their first "deep thought" was. (Journaling is a great tool for remembering these things later on!)

Because cannabis helps us to see things from a viewpoint outside of ourselves, it does indeed give us a "higher" knowledge. We can look "down" at the situation now and see it from a "higher," more omniscient view. This gives us more information to help resolve issues, boost creativity, and find new and better ways to complete a task.

What task, issue, or situation in your life could use a second pair of eyes? A pair of eyes with an excellent view? Meditate on it today to see your issue from a new viewpoint.

August 27

Serenity

Bring serenity into your world today with a calm, relaxing meditation. Visualize yourself in an environment that fulfills your requirements for pure relaxation. Let your mind be at ease. Let it rest. Allow all troubles and thoughts to fall away.

This time is for you and you alone.

At one.

At peace.

August 28

Trance dance

Our harvests have begun, both literal and metaphysical—it is time to celebrate the bounty of the earth and the work we have achieved so far. It is the season of giving thanks, so give thanks in dance with a song that makes you want to celebrate the earth and her abundance along with your own accomplishments.

I prefer to use "Soles on Earth" by Zingaia.

When you are ready, begin moving with the music. Block out everything but the sound of the music.

If physical limitations require it, remain seated while moving to the music.

You can "dance" with whatever body parts you want to use. Feel free to move in whatever way feels the most pleasing to you.

Allow the music to wash over and consume you.

Where does it take you?

August 29

Chant

"Sun above me,
earth below me,
guide me to be
strong."

This is an easy-to-remember chant to help you connect with both the grounding energy of the earth below you and the strength of the sun above. While the sun is scorching and we feel the strongest effects of his rays, it's a good time to absorb some of that energy for ourselves.

Do this chant where you can feel the sun shine down on your face.

Repeat this chant throughout your meditation.

Try saying it in different intonations and at different speeds until you find your match.

How does this chant make you feel?

What does it mean to you?

August 30
Visualized quest

Go on a visualized personal quest today—a journey deep into the oneness with the universe—to see what spirits have a message for you. Shut all other thoughts out of your mind and pay attention to what and who comes to visit with you. What do you see? Hear? Smell? Reach out with your senses and open yourself to the message.

August 31
Breathwork

Take time in this month's breathwork to lose your breath.

How do you lose your breath?

Best way I can think of is to laugh yourself silly.

Adjust your dose from "meditative" to "giggle fit" and think of the funniest moments of your life. Once you start going, you know it will continue for a while, and the more you try to tamper down those giggles, the more they will creep up on you, so just let them out and enjoy.

Enjoy the workout laughter gives you.

Afterwards, take a few deep calming breaths to help center and ground.

❈ SEPTEMBER SHOPPING LIST ❈

Lapis lazuli (September 9)

Dried crushed anise (September 15)

Grapes (at least 3 varieties) (September 20)

Gardenia essential oil (September 29)

September 1
Reflection

Reflection can bring both joy and sorrow, sometimes at the same time. Let the cannabis guide you today to a moment you need to reflect upon—whether it be a happy moment or a painful moment, simply let whatever comes to mind play out. Don't force a memory. The one you need to revisit, the one you need to see, will come to you. Reflect on the memory with new eyes, with eyes removed from the situation. What lesson does this reflection have for you today?

September 2
Dreamtime

There is nothing wrong with a little daydreaming, and cannabis is a great booster to get those creative juices flowing to ferry you away into dreamland. Meditate on a happy place today. It may be real or imaginary. What does it look like? Who is with you? (It's your dream so you can include whoever or whatever you want.) What are you all doing? Allow the scenario to play out. Revel in the joy the dream brings to you.

September 3
The ripening

It's getting closer to the dark part of the year. More crops are ripening every day. The days are growing shorter and soon will be equal to the night. Step back and watch as the wheel of time slowly turns. We must turn with it as our thoughts and exploits turn from outward work to finishing up projects bringing in our harvest. Feel your energy adjust to the energy around you; the dog days of summer are replaced with the quickening of running out of daylight. Plants put their efforts into growing and ripening fruits instead of growing the vines that support them. Turn your energy to ripening your own fruits.

September 4
Enlightenment

Every time your soul learns something new, you have attained a new level of enlightenment. You have taken a step toward healing your soul. Cannabis is a great aid in the quest for enlightenment due to the effects it has on our psyche—when we allow it to. Your soul can tell you where it needs healing, where the lessons are that need to be learned, you simply must listen to what it has to say.

Listen to your soul in today's meditation. What message does it have for you? What do you need to heal?

September 5
Hope

Hope is the building block of our dreams. It is what motivates us to try and to succeed. When hope runs out, we fail.

Meditate today on a time when you gave up hope. Why did you lose it? What was the outcome? Look back on the event objectively. Do you need to reassess the situation and build hope again, or have your dreams changed for the better?

September 6
Delight

Think back to when you were a young child. What is something that brought you pure delight? Something that made you giddy with happiness? Do you still get that feeling in your life? Do you feel joy and delight at the same level as you did as a child, or has part of that faded away? We seem to lose pure delight as we get older. Meditate today on those things that brought you such complete happiness. How can you bring that same happiness into your life today?

September 7
Raise your vibration

This term is used so often, yet it is not always defined in terms people easily comprehend, especially if you are new to the term.

Picture this.

Negativity bogs you down. It slows you down and makes you feel heavy and lethargic.

Positivity has the opposite effect. It gives you energy and a natural "high."

Raising your vibration, simply put, means ridding your body, mind, and spirit of some negativity, and replacing it with positivity.

Meditate on the negativity you need to remove from your life. What can you toss out to raise your vibration? Rid yourself of negativity and grab a refill of positivity to go.

September 8
Shine your light

The world would be a much brighter place if we all would turn on our inner light and let it shine for everyone to see. Meditate today on what you can do to show your inner light to the world around you. How would it feel to live in a world where this was the norm?

September 9
Get stoned: lapis lazuli

Lapis lazuli is used to increase physic awareness, help relieve depression, and deals with all aspects of healing—spiritually, emotionally, mentally, and physically. It is an ideal stone to wear daily for someone struggling on their path. It is uplifting.

Choose one or more of these qualities that calls to you. Which of these aspects do you need most in your life, and what can you combine together to charge your stone perfectly for your purposes?

Get into your comfy spot and hold the stone in your hand out in front of you.

Examine the stone with your eyes and your fingers.

Feel the stone as you hold it tightly in your hand.

Hold the stone close to your heart.

Meditate on the stone and how it feels to you.

Carry this stone with you whenever you feel the need.

September 10
Call of the wild: swamp sounds

Do an online search for "swamp sounds."

Find a clip that is a good length for your meditation time or use a repeat feature.

Play the clip and meditate on it as you listen.

Do you like this sound? Dislike the sound?

Let the sound encompass you.
How does it make you feel?

September 11
In memorial

If you were old enough, you probably remember right where you were and what you were doing the day the United States sustained a terrible terrorist attack. Even if you weren't alive yet or don't remember, you know the events of the day.

During your meditation, pay honor, respect, and remembrance to those souls lost.

September 12
Signs and symbols

One of the benefits of cannabis is the way it opens your mind to see things you may otherwise miss. Minute details become bolder under the influence of cannabis. These details often contain signs or symbols that get overlooked in daily life. Use today's meditation to commit to looking for the signs and symbols in your day-to-day life. Often what you need the most is right under your own nose; you just have to be able to see it. Where are the signs pointing you? What symbols have been trying to get your attention? Combine these concepts together to find your full picture.

September 13
Primal instincts

Cannabis lowers your inhibitions and allows you to shut off your filter. It also encourages other primal instincts, sex included!

In today's meditation, put on some music of your choice and move to it with a primal instincts attitude. Let your body tell the story it wants. Don't think, just move. Close your eyes if you are in a location where it is safe to without bumping into things or falling.

September 14
Natural relief

Depending on where you live, true fall may soon be on the way. Cooler temperatures, blustery days, torrential rain, and snow all tend to keep people inside, so if you can perform today's meditation outside, do so. If not, perform your meditation near an open window.

Nature helps rejuvenate ourselves—body, mind and spirit. The fresh air and sunshine help us physically as well as helping to clear our minds and lift our spirits. Meditate today in nature while focusing on how being in nature helps you to heal.

Visualize fresh air entering your lungs in a cleansing white light. The oxygen from the air absorbs into your blood and is carried throughout your body by your veins, the cleansing white light traveling with it as it goes.

The sun shines down on you, warming you, enriching your skin with vitamin D.

Allow the breeze to carry away your burdens, to lighten your load for now.

Let the natural world reach through and heal you.

September 15
Smoke the herb: anise
Anise corresponds to purification and protection.

Combine your cannabis with some dried ground anise. Use a mix of about 90 percent cannabis to 10 percent anise, but you can adjust that according to your preferences.

When combining herbs with cannabis for the first time, always resort back to "slow and low." You are introducing a new combination of acids, proteins, and terpenes to your system. Give yourself time to see how it affects you, and that's all you have to do. Meditate on your reactions: How does it make you feel? Do you like it? How can you use this combination further in your practices?

September 16
Chill lounge
Change is coming. It is imminent. The growth cycle is slowing, shifting towards rest. The leaves of the trees begin to

change colors for their grand finale before the curtain falls. We, too, need to finish up our projects. It is last call for the summer. Last call for the outer work we do before focusing our work inward.

Choose a song that reflects this theme for you—this shift in nature, time, and energy.

I prefer to use "New Camelot" by Llewellyn.

Play your music while you are in your comfy spot. Let not only the music but any lyrics flow over you, and listen deeply and intently. Where does the music take you? How does it make you feel?

September 17

Knee high to a grasshopper

We've all heard this exaggeration, and there have even been a few movies made about people being shrunk down to the tiniest size, where riding on ants is possible.

But what if it was possible?

Have some fun in your meditation time today. Imagine what life would be like if you were knee high to a grasshopper. What would your home be made from? What would you eat? Take an adventure into the wild, but in an extremely miniature size.

September 18
Inner witness

Your conscious is your inner witness. It sees all, hears all, knows all. In your meditation today, let your inner witness come through and show you some of your not-so proud moments. While you cannot undo these moments, you can learn from them. What does your inner witness want you to know?

September 19
Hearth and home

Give thanks today for your home and those who are closest to you. Spend time in deep appreciation for what you have. We are often more willing to complain than we are to appreciate and praise, so be very specific and conscious of what you are giving thanks for. Remind yourself how lucky you are to have the life you do instead of something far worse. Be aware of your blessings.

September 20
Got the munchies: grapes

After dosing, get into your comfy spot and set a bowl of grapes right by you. Have three different varieties of grapes. This meditation is going to focus on your taste buds and other sensations. Keep your eyes closed so that you are not relying on your sense of sight. Use your sense of smell to take in the scent of each grape before you eat it. Can you identify it from the scent? (That would be incredible!) Pay extreme attention to what you are doing as you take a bite. Feel your teeth sink into the grape. Experience the textures and flavor, singling them out as much as possible. Take your time and enjoy each of the grapes, testing yourself to see if you can identify each one by the taste and texture. Use this type of meditation anytime you are eating for a fuller, richer connection with your food. Feel free to add music to make your meditation more intense.

September 21
Make an offering

Start the new season off with an offering. It does not have to be a physical offering but an offering from your heart, mind, or spirit. Give this offering to your deities, your higher power, or the universe at large.

For physical offerings, now is the perfect time if you do any vegetable gardening to offer some of your harvest.

This is also a good time to do volunteer work in areas that help deal with transitions or in preparing things for the winter to come. This can be anything from working with the homeless to cleaning up trash along roadways or public areas before the leaves begin covering them as they fall.

Meditate on what offerings you have to give.

September 22
Shifting the balance

The balance is shifting; the days will now be shorter than the nights. The leaves stop collecting sunlight to convert to energy and instead dry up and fall off. The fields begin going fallow. The end of the harvest is close at hand. It is time for us to begin shifting our own balance. We become more internal, shifting our focus from producing energy to harvesting our goals and preparing to go fallow for the winter.

Visualize yourself as a tree. Your leaves have lost their chlorophyll; they no longer gather sunlight. The days grow darker and colder. The wind blows your leaves away. You cocoon into a deep slumber. Know it is time for you to listen to the lesson of the trees and prepare for your own time of rest.

September 23
Go with the flow

This meditation is great to do outside, especially if you can safely do it near a body of water, particularly a river, creek, or stream. If not possible, simply visualize that is where you are. Listen to the sound of the water flowing next to your ear. Relax and let yourself feel as if you are floating on the water, going with the flow; at times, the water splashes over you, cooling you where the sun has been warming your skin. Let the water wash away your worries, stress, any problems. For the here and now, it is just you, relaxing, floating, weightless.

September 24
Power

Some people crave it, some people are afraid of it. What is your relationship with power? Are you comfortable with your own power? Today in your meditation, focus on it. See yourself in control of your power—using it for good, not harm, not encroaching on others' power. Remind yourself you have all the strength and power you need; it is already within you.

September 25
Exploration

Take off into the universe of oneness with your high. While you do not have to hit a peak experience, if you can, go ahead! Explore the universe around you: What does it look like? How do you feel? Explore all around you. This oneness, as you see it, is your own creation, and yet it may feel new and foreign to you. Whatever you encounter in your universe has a message for you. Bring the message back with you.

September 26
Inspirational inklings

"...as more individuals learn to identify, cultivate, and pro-long peak experiences, we stand to witness considerable social betterment, given that human society is ultimately a set of relationships, the quality of which reflect our inner selves. Therefore when more of us become aware of the temporal and the eternal realms of consciousness, then to resolve tensions and conflicts, we may choose the avenue for dialogue rather than belligerence."

—Mark S. Ferrara[16]

According to Ferrara, peak experiences can help us improve not only our relationships but learn to end conflict by opening up dialogues. How have your experiences improved your relationships? How have you been able to open better dialogues?

September 27
Chant

"I am peace.
I am love.
I am hope.
I am strong."

---

16. Mark S. Ferrara, *Sacred Bliss: A Spiritual History of Cannabis* (Lanham, MD: Rowman & Littlefield, 2016), 101.

Enjoy this simple peace, love, hippie type of chant. Allow it to lift your spirit and let it soar.

Repeat this chant throughout your meditation. Feel free to add a drum or other percussion instrument such as a rattle.

Try saying it in different intonations and at different speeds until you find your match.

How does this chant make you feel?

What does it mean to you?

September 28

Trance dance

Once again, as the seasons change and the energies shift, so do we. It is a wonderful time to be able to be outside, knowing the days are growing shorter and the nights longer; the cold, dark of winter is on the way. Our energies will soon be turning from the outer workings to inner workings but, like the leaves on the trees, we can put on a beautiful show. Take advantage of these days to perform your trance dance outside if possible.

Look for a song that speaks of nature to you. A song that sings of harvests, a change of seasons, and a shift in energies.

I use "Enter the Sacred" by David and Steve Gordon.

When you are ready, begin moving with the music. Block out everything but the sound of the music.

If physical limitations require it, remain seated while moving to the music.

You can "dance" with whatever body parts you want to use. Feel free to move in whatever way feels the most pleasing to you.

Allow the music to wash over and consume you.

Where does it take you?

September 29
Breathe it in: gardenia oil

Gardenia is used to attract love and peace. It helps a heart heal and increases spiritual connections, making it extremely beneficial for peak experiences.

Decide your purpose for working with the oil. Choose what correspondence(s) you want to focus on for this session. Since it does increase spiritual connections, this is always an excellent choice if you want to open yourself to receive whatever message it is you need to hear.

Prepare your meditation area ahead of time. You may want to use a diffuser to which you can add a few drops of oil. Use a self-lighting charcoal tablet in a fireproof container, and once the tablet is lit, add a few drops of oil to it for an intense burst of the scent. If you want to use the oil on your skin, be sure to add it to a carrier oil first. To keep it simple, sniff the oil from the bottle.

Use the oil in your chosen method. Close your eyes and inhale the scent deeply and slowly several times before allowing yourself to breathe normally again. Immerse yourself in the scent so that you feel its aura all around you. If you need to, take more slow, deep breaths to increase the intensity of the scent.

What feelings does this scent invoke in you? Does it bring back memories? Do you have a connection to this scent?

Feel free to add music to this meditation.

September 30
Breathwork
Reflect over the month with breaths of gratitude. With each breathing cycle you make—inhalation, hold, exhalation—recall a moment of gratitude from the past month to acknowledge it once again. Once you have cycled through the month, run back through it again. This time look for moments where you missed acknowledging your gratitude at the time. What sticks out to you that you missed? Acknowledge it now. Continue breathing in your gratitude for as long as you like.

✳ OCTOBER SHOPPING LIST ✳

Tourmaline (October 11)

Pomegranate (October 21)

Cinnamon essential oil (October 27)

Dried crushed mugwort (October 28)

October 1
Intuition

Intuition—the little voice inside your head that lets you know things simply by letting you know them. There is no independent thought or reasoning. The information is just there. We all have the ability for intuition; it's more a matter of whether we allow it to come through and if we listen to it. Evaluate how well your intuition is developed. Do you use it often? Do you have blockages or walls preventing efficient use? How best does your intuition serve you?

October 2
Inspirational inklings

"You've got to know yourself so that you can at last *be* yourself."

—D.H. Lawrence[17]

---

17. D. H. Lawrence, *The Collected Works of D. H. Lawrence* (Hastings, UK: Delphi Classics, 2015), n.p.

Getting to know yourself can be difficult and, most likely, what you think you know, isn't the full story. We live with a psyche that can be activated to protect us, even from ourselves. It takes breaking down our own walls to dive in deep enough to get to know the real you. The upside, of course, is once you know who you are—you can be who you are.

How has cannabis helped you to break down walls to help you discover who you are?

October 3

Sacred space

October is a magical time as the veil between our world and the otherworld thins. It is a time when we honor our ancestors and mourn those we have lost. It is the time of the final harvest. For some spiritual practices, it is the end of the year. Halloween is often seen now as a "season" instead of just one day. It is when we truly feel the onset of the dark half of the year. It is a sacred space in time. Meditate on what this sacred space means to you. Do you feel the magic in the air? The thinning of the veil? Do you hear your ancestors calling out to you?

October 4
Ancient wisdom

Ancient wisdom from our ancestors may feel like it is lost to us, but it doesn't have to be. We can use our connection to the universe to listen to their stories and lessons. They are here to teach us if we are willing to hear them. Using cannabis to hit a peak experience is a beautiful and effective way to connect to the universe to absorb the wisdom of your ancestors. If you cannot hit a peak, that is okay. Still, open your mind and focus on hearing from those who existed generations before. What do they have to teach you?

October 5
Honor your ancestors

It is incredible to think of all the people who had to exist in order for us to be here today. We carry the DNA of hundreds of people, being passed down from generation to generation. They are a part of each one of us. In today's meditation, think about and honor these people. Think of the choices they made, which eventually led to your existence. Thank them for contributing to who you are today.

October 6
Into the mystic

Let today's meditation take you to a place of mystical magic—whatever that means for you. Whether it be the magical shores of Avalon or to the Shire of Middle Earth, go to a place real or imaginary where you feel magic all around you. Visualize what life would be like living in this mystical location.

October 7
Your tribe

Your tribe is your closest family and friends. The people who help you survive. The people you count on and who know you have their back. You have a symbiotic relationship with them. Often, these people are a part of your spiritual family. Think about who is in your tribe. You have probably lost tribe members over the years due to death or other circumstances. Say a solemn thank you and goodbye to those now gone. Give thanks for those who are still with you.

October 8
Confront your fears

Confronting your fears in meditation is an excellent way to begin working through them and learning how to tolerate them, if not get rid of them all together. What fears do you have? Meditate on one fear today. Step outside of yourself for an objective view on where your fear came from. Knowing the root of a fear is a leap toward overcoming it. Listen to the universe for suggestions on coping with and ending this fear.

October 9
Kindred spirits
Your kindred spirits are those people who have some of the same interests as you. Spiritually, they may be souls you have encountered in other incarnations, in other lifetimes. These are the people that, when you meet them, you feel an instant connection, as if you had already met somewhere before. It can feel more like a reunion than a chance meeting. Who are your kindred spirits in your life? Meditate on your relationships with them. Can you feel a spiritual connection to any of them from a different time? Allow yourself to be guided by your higher consciousness to view your relationships in other lives.

October 10
Call of the wild: wind blowing through the trees
Do an online search for "wind blowing through trees."

Find a clip that is a good length for your meditation time or use a repeat feature.

Play the clip and meditate on it as you listen.

Let the sound encompass you.
Do you like this sound? Dislike the sound?
How does it make you feel?

October 11
Get stoned: tourmaline

Tourmaline is a multicolored stone that resonates with healing, love, friendship, peace, sleep, energy, courage, inspiration, protection, and matters relating to business.

Choose one or more of these qualities that calls to you. What do you need to call into your life? How can you combine traits to charge a stone unique for you? Are you starting a new business venture or career? Energy, courage, inspiration, protection wrapped up together with tourmaline's ability to deal with business matters would make this ideal to have around to help you settle in. Tourmaline can work with the more emotional side as well, assisting with healing, friendships, love, and peace.

Get into your comfy spot and hold the stone in your hand out in front of you.

Examine the stone with your eyes and your fingers.

Feel the stone as you hold it tightly in your hand.

Hold the stone close to your heart.

Meditate on the stone and how it feels to you.

Carry this stone with you whenever you feel the need.

October 12
Respect

The people we respect, those we deeply admire and hold in high regard, have an extreme effect on our lives. They help to shape who we are. We want to emulate them. We want to live up to their ideals and standards. Who in your life has earned this type of respect? Why do you respect them? How has this person(s) shaped who you are? What qualities of theirs do you want to emulate in your life?

October 13
Mystery

October is filled with mystery, magic, and sometimes a little bit of mayhem. Think back to the way Halloween was celebrated many years ago, with carved turnips and people dressed in costume to ward off ghosts and other evil spirits. Let yourself travel back in time to dance around a bonfire. Summer has ended, the last of the harvests are coming in, the flocks are being culled to salt for winter storage. Spend your meditation visiting this land and time from which Halloween was born.

October 14
Chill lounge

Honor the energies of nature as we accept death is a part of every life. We honor life by honoring death. We honor death by honoring life. Energy transfers from one form to another. The cycle continues, the circle unbroken.

Choose a song that honors the importance of death as a form of energy transference. A song that allows you to feel pride, loss, and hope for a renewal.

I enjoy "Samhain" by Trobar de Morte.

Play your music while you are in your comfy spot. Let not only the music but any lyrics flow over you, and listen deeply and intently. Where does the music take you? How does it make you feel?

October 15

Former lives

With October's connection to the past and ancestors, it is also a perfect time to delve into your former lives.

Reach back into the past with your mind. Is there a time period you are drawn to? How does it make you feel? Sad? Happy? Allow a specific time to come through to you. Let it surround you and take you there. Focus on who you may have been in this time period. Allow the images, thoughts, feelings to come to you. Allow the universe to guide you and to introduce you to a former version of your spirit. What soul lesson did your spirit learn in that incarnation? Does your past self have any advice or message for your current self?

October 16
A blustery day
You know that feeling you get when it's cold and rainy outside but you are warm and toasty inside with your thick fleece socks, bowl of hot soup, and the best blanket in the world? Maybe your ideal of cozy takes place next to a fireplace or in a bean bag or your favorite chair. Wherever your "let the world do what it wants out there because I am safe in here" spot is, go there. Meditate on being in that situation. Outside is nasty terrible (whether it is or not, imagine it is), but you are snug inside. Blissful. Thankfully enjoying your comfort.

October 17
Coming to an end
As we delve deeper into the dark half of the year, your goals and projects should be wrapping up with completion. It will soon be the time for rest and to turn our thoughts and workings internal once again. Meditate today on all you have accomplished in this cycle. Give yourself a virtual pat on the back. Feel pride in the work you have done. You deserve it.

October 18

Absence makes the heart grow fonder

While it is true for some people that "out of sight means out of mind," for others, absence truly does make the heart grow fonder. This is especially true with those we have loved and lost. Their absence helps to erase negative memories, letting the positive ones hold on longer and stronger. Our memories of the person become more loving, and indeed we grow fonder. Moments of anger and sadness involving our loved one are replaced with happiness and love.

Meditate today on some of your fondest memories of a love lost. While these memories may still bring sadness at the loss, focus on the joy of their remembrance.

October 19

Slamming doors

When a door closes in our lives, it doesn't always mean a window opens. Sometimes it is a harsh, unexpected, slam in the face. A slamming door is a sudden, unexpected major loss—this may be in the form of a death, a terminated job, the loss of a long-term or committed relationship. They are events beyond our control. Actions we could not prevent, decisions made by others without our input. A slamming door leaves us powerless, at least temporarily.

What slamming doors have you had to deal with in your life? How did you deal with it? Meditate today on how you reacted. How do you regain your power after a door is slammed in your face?

October 20
Tying up loose ends

Have you completed all your goals for the year? Have all your plans come to fruition? Do you still have loose ends to tie up to finish certain tasks? Evaluate where you are on everything today. What steps do you need to take to finish up anything left? Set your plans in your mind. Visualize what you need to do, and see yourself as being successful in all that you want to achieve but haven't yet.

October 21
Got the munchies: pomegranate

After dosing, get into your comfy spot and set a bowl of pomegranate seeds right by you. (Keep in mind that pomegranate juice stains can be hard to get out, so choose a location and clothes you're okay with getting stained.) This meditation is going to focus on your taste buds and other sensations. Keep your eyes closed so that you are not relying on your sense of sight. Use your sense of smell to take in the scent of each seed before you eat it. Pay extreme attention to what you are doing as you take a bite.

Feel your teeth sink through the skin of the pomegranate flesh. Experience the textures and flavor, singling them out as much as possible. Take your time and enjoy each of the seeds. Use this type of meditation anytime you are eating for a fuller, richer connection with your food.

October 22
Veiled fog

For a bit of a spooky touch to this meditation, perform it outside in the dark—especially if you are blessed with a foggy night!

Fog is mystical (small pun intended). It brings to mind a barrier between worlds, such as the famous mists surrounding Avalon of Arthurian legend. In October, on a cool fall night, when the veil thins more with each passing day, fog can feel like a gateway into another world. So why not use it?

Find yourself deep in thick fog swirling and whirling around you. It's your fog, so be as creative as you want with it, make it the whitest white, or a variety of colors, weaving in and out of each other like tentacles.

Let the fog consume you for as long as you like. When ready for the fog to lift, let it reveal something to you. What do you find?

October 23
Inspirational inklings

"It really puzzles me to see marijuana connected with narcotics, dope, and all of that stuff. It is a thousand times better than whiskey. It is an assistant and a friend."

—Louis Armstrong[18]

The world-famous jazz musician Louis Armstrong used "gage" throughout much of his career and credited it with helping him to create much of his music. How has cannabis been an assistant to you? How has it been a friend?

October 24
Enchantment

Enchanter. Sorcerer. Witch. Let today's meditation take you into a world of magic. What powers do you have? What enchantments would you cast? Visualize yourself as whatever type of great magician you wish. Let your imagination take you where it will.

---

18. Callie Barrons, "25 Inspirational Quotes About Weed," High Times, June 22, 2018, https://hightimes.com/culture/inspirational -quotes-about-weed/8/.

October 25

Trance dance

There is something about drum music on a chilled October night, particularly if you have the joy of being able to have some sort of campfire or bonfire close by. This may be your last chance to get outside for a trance dance due to weather, so if you can, always feel free to head outdoors for your time in the zone.

Drums are lively. They are uplifting. With the natural world around us taking on the semblance of death, we must remember it is only going to rest for a while. In all endings are new beginnings, and those beginnings will be here soon enough.

Choose a song with a lot of drums or a fast drumbeat —a song you can really move with to raise energy.

As soon as I discovered "Trance Dance Drum Journey with Throat Singing" by Project for Gaia, I knew it was the perfect song for me to do this meditation with.

When you are ready, begin moving with the music. Block out everything but the sound of the music.

If physical limitations require it, remain seated while moving to the music.

You can "dance" with whatever body parts you want to use. Feel free to move in whatever way feels the most pleasing to you.

Allow the music to wash over and consume you.

Where does it take you?

October 26
Trick or Treat?

If we are lucky, there is still a bit of a child hidden deep inside of us. Someone who loves to play, have fun, and perhaps, when the time is right, conjure up a little mischief. Think back to your childhood memories. Did you participate in the tradition of trick or treating? What are your memories like? Did your memories live up to your expectations? Let your imagination whisk you away into your ultimate world of trick or treat.

October 27
Breathe it in: cinnamon oil

Cinnamon is a versatile oil used for energy, psychic awareness, power and success, and love and lust.

Decide your purpose for working with the oil. Choose what correspondence(s) you want to focus on for this session. Whether you want to use it to boost your psychic awareness for divination or spirit communication, you are looking for a boost in your romantic life, or are up for a promotion at work, you can combine different qualities to create what works best for your situation.

Prepare your meditation area ahead of time. You may want to use a diffuser to which you can add a few drops of oil. Use a self-lighting charcoal tablet in a fireproof container, and once the tablet is lit, add a few drops of oil to it for an intense burst of the scent. If you want to use the oil on your skin, be sure to add it to a carrier oil first. To keep it simple, sniff the oil from the bottle.

Use the oil in your chosen method. Close your eyes and inhale the scent deeply and slowly several times before allowing yourself to breathe normally again. Immerse yourself in the scent so that you feel its aura all around you. If you need to, take more slow, deep breaths to increase the intensity of the scent.

What feelings does this scent invoke in you? Does it bring back memories? Do you have a connection to this scent?

Feel free to add music to this meditation.

October 28
Smoke the herb: mugwort
Mugwort is a great herb in the metaphysical world for how it increases psychic powers. It is used to bring on dreams and aid in divination, clairvoyance, and astral projection. It is also used for protection and to boost strength.

Combine your cannabis with some dried ground mugwort. I use a mix of about 70 percent cannabis to 30 percent herb, but you can adjust that according to your preferences.

When combining herbs with cannabis for the first time, always resort back to "slow and low." You are introducing a new combination of acids, proteins, and terpenes to your system. Give yourself time to see how it affects you, and that's all you have to do. Meditate on your reactions: How does it make you feel? Do you like it? How can you use this combination further in your practices?

October 29
Chant
"The days grow short.
The nights grow cold.
Memories turn
to thoughts of old."

Designed to set you in the spirit of remembrance, with memories both good and bad, use this chant to help you reflect on your life, particularly on the changes and choices that have made you who you are today. Think back to your defining moments and the path you have chosen. Do not question it, simply remember. You are precisely where you need to be.

Repeat this chant throughout your meditation.

Try saying it in different intonations and at different speeds until you find your match.

How does this chant make you feel? Let it bring out memories you need to be reminded of. Look at them with new eyes; is there a message for you?

October 30
Breathwork

For this month's breathwork, focus on slowing down.

Begin by breathing normally. Pay attention to your normal breath. Follow the rise and fall of your chest and abdomen. Consciously slow your breathing down slightly. Try not to count out your inhalations and exhalations, instead, hyper focus on how the speed feels to you. Once you feel yourself slow it, hold it for several breath cycles until you are ready to slow it down again. The sensation becomes almost hypnotic. Continue to see how much you can comfortably slow it down. Continue as long as you wish.

October 31
Commune with your ancestors

The veil is at its thinnest, so it is the perfect time to reach out in your meditation to your ancestors long gone—the hundreds, the thousands of people who had to exist in order for you to be you. Here, today. Without all of them, you would not be the person you are. Reach out to your ancestors. Thank them for the choices they made that brought about your existence. Thank them for the DNA handed down for generations. You share primal building blocks with these people. They are your family, your kin. Ask for any messages they may have for you.

✳ NOVEMBER SHOPPING LIST ✳

Citrine (November 10)

Fresh pears—at least 2 varieties, 3 if you can find them (November 20)

Nutmeg essential oil (November 27)

Ground clove (November 28)

November 1
Legends

Whether fictional characters or historical persons, legends inspire us. They are larger than life. Their flaws appear minimal because the best of their character is what survives in the telling of their heroic stories. What legends have you looked up to in your life? What about their personality and character do you admire? How has this legend inspired you in your life?

November 2
Ethics

Your ethics are your own personal code of conduct. The do's and don'ts of your life. As you age and mature, your code of conduct changes and evolves. Evaluate your ethics today. How have they changed over your lifetime? Do you live up to your own code?

November 3
Misunderstandings

Texts, emails, social media, messaging apps. All these newer forms of communications have added a mass of confusion and misunderstandings to our world. We jump to conclusions on what someone's intent was behind a typed message when we can't hear their voice, tone, and inflection. We can't see their facial expressions, their body language, nothing but their words, and we misinterpret the few clues we have. Think about a time when a typed communication brought with it a misunderstanding for you. How did you deal with it? What can you learn from how you dealt with it? How can you prevent misunderstandings in the future?

November 4
Generosity

This is the time of year when charities send out their annual appeals. Food drives, coat drives, adopt-a-child for holiday presents drives, they are everywhere. Charities must count on the generosity of others at this time of year to fulfill the needs of their clients. While people do tend to feel more generous at the holidays, the problem is that people do not tend to feel more generous throughout the entire year. Evaluate your own generosity today. Could you be more generous with your talent? Time? Money?

Think about ways you can show generosity year-round, not only at the holidays.

November 5
Please forgive me

Sometimes, we are the villain in someone else's story—whether we mean to be or not. We can ask for forgiveness, yet it doesn't mean we will get it.

How do you go on when forgiveness isn't given?

Use this meditation to reflect on forgiveness you sought but never received. Try to put yourself in the other person's shoes. Do you understand why they were unable to forgive? How did your actions affect them?

Even if you would have acted differently to the same behavior, set that aside. This is about how someone else feels, not you.

Actions have consequences, and sometimes those consequences are difficult to accept. When forgiveness is not given, it can make accepting those consequences even more difficult.

What have you learned from your experience? People come and go from our lives. They teach us lessons about ourselves and help us to grow even if they don't stick around. Use what you have learned to build empathy for others and to respect their feelings and choices.

November 6
Appreciation

It truly feels wonderful to be appreciated. It makes our hearts happy and we glow. You know what else feels wonderful and makes your heart happy and your soul glow? Appreciating others. Appreciating life. Appreciating beauty. Appreciating love.

Meditate today on how well you show appreciation to and for others. Do you do it enough? Do you go overboard so much it doesn't come off as sincere? Contemplate on ways you can show your appreciation more in the future.

November 7
Self-care

Make today a self-care day. In your meditation, check in with your body. Are you holding stress or other negativities in your muscles? Allow yourself to fully relax and take a conscious break for yourself. Let yourself unwind and put aside all thoughts but those of comfort and peace. Give yourself time to relax and take time for you. You deserve it.

November 8
Compassion

The winter months, the dark half of the year, are traditionally a time of introspection. We work on the inside and face our own darkness in preparation to bloom in the spring. One of the areas we need to explore is compassion—compassion for others as well as compassion for ourselves.

Compassion is not only about feeling sympathy for others—true compassion includes the desire to end suffering. We often forget about this second part, the desire to end suffering. In some people, it is an overwhelming need to end the suffering of others.

Where in your life and environment do you feel compassion?

Where in your life and environment are you lacking compassion?

What changes can you make to alleviate your own suffering or the suffering of others?

November 9
Call of the wild: ocean waves

Do an online search for "ocean waves sound."

Find a clip that is a good length for your meditation time or use a repeat feature.

Play the clip and meditate on it as you listen.

Do you like this sound? Dislike the sound?
Let the sound encompass you.
How does it make you feel?

November 10
Get stoned: citrine

Citrine is a yellow stone that resonates with joy, creativity, communication, psychic powers, and sexual energy, and it helps to prevent nightmares.

Choose one or more of these qualities that calls to you. Which of these things do you need to bring into your life? What creative ways can you combine qualities to specialize a stone for you? If you have nightmares, focus on turning your dreams into communication devices that hone your psychic powers to bring you messages of joy and creativity instead. Discover how it can work for you.

Get into your comfy spot and hold the stone in your hand out in front of you.

Examine the stone with your eyes and your fingers.
Feel the stone as you hold it tightly in your hand.
Hold the stone close to your heart.
Meditate on the stone and how it feels to you.
Carry this stone with you whenever you feel the need.

November 11

Connection

Holidays bring people together. People you want to be with, and sometimes people you really do not want to be with. At all. Remind yourself, we are all in this crazy rat race together. We are all together. We are one. Today, reach out to your connection to one, your connection to the universe. No matter how different people are, no matter how people feel about one another, there is one thing we all have in common: We are all here. We are all together. We are one.

November 12

It's not the time

Being with family at the holidays can be bittersweet. For some people, it brings up past issues that have never fully healed. Remember—it's not the time.

It's not the time to doubt yourself. It's not the time to let others put you down or insult you in a failed attempt to make up for their own shortcomings. It's not the time to put yourself into debt to prove your love to someone. It's not the time to allow others to answer for you. It's not the time to hide who you are to make others comfortable. It is not the time to give in to the expectations of others at your own cost. Spend time in meditation today telling yourself what it is not the time for and put away those familial roles you have played in the past.

November 13
Inner sanctuary
Step into your inner sanctuary today. Check in with your body, mind, and spirit. Send white light energy to any areas of your body in need of healing. Relax your body and mind and allow your spirit to soar.

November 14
Fate
What are your views on fate? Do you believe everything is planned out for us and we are pawns in someone else's game? Do you believe we have free will and every decision we make is our own and leads us down a new path? Or do your beliefs on fate meld together somewhere in between? Meditate today on your idea of fate. What control do you believe you have? What do you believe is beyond your control and fated instead?

November 15
Inspirational inklings

"As human beings, our greatness lies not so much in being able to remake the world … as in being able to remake ourselves."

—Mahatma Gandhi[19]

We often want the world to be a better place. We want to change everything to the way we think would be best. What would be best for us. But what is best for us may not be what is best for other people. This is hard to accept, but it's also a very valid reason as to why instead of trying to remake the world around us, we need to remake ourselves to be the best we can be. If everyone made remade themselves into the best they could be, the world would automatically change along with it.

How have you already been remaking yourself? What work do you have to do?

November 16
Chill lounge

The end of fall. The trees are bare. The fields are fallow. The outside world appears to be covered in death. But

---

19. Viral Mehta, "Lessons in Living on the Edge From Mahatma Gandhi," Huffpost, August 31, 2011, https://www.huffpost.com/entry/selfless-action_b_940035.

below the surface, life survives, at rest. It is a time of letting go of what is beyond our control and what no longer serves us. It is a time to be thankful for what we have. It is a time of hope for things to come.

What song helps incorporate these emotions for you?

I use "Life and Death" by Paul Cardall.

Play your music while you are in your comfy spot. Let not only the music but any lyrics flow over you, and listen deeply and intently. Where does the music take you? How does it make you feel?

November 17

Pleasure

Allow yourself a bit of pleasure in today's meditation in whatever form you wish. Focus on something that brings you great joy. Give yourself a bit of indulgent fun. This may include a sensual dance, giving yourself a massage with cannabis-infused oil, or a special treat of cannabis-infused chocolate. Perhaps you simply want to visualize lying on a beach, swimming in a hidden lagoon, or relaxing in a meadow of wildflowers. Whatever will bring you pleasure at this moment, go there today.

November 18
Crossroads

Difficult decisions. Different pathways. Each one taking you to a completely different destination, not to mention the significant individual encounters along the way. How do you choose? How do you know which way to go? What is the process you used to decide which pathway to take? Does it tend to work for you, or do you often find yourself in regret? What lessons have you learned from your times at a crossroad?

November 19
Feeling whole

You do not need any other human to complete you. You are your own full, whole person. You do not need to find "your other half." You are not split into two. All your pieces are there, hidden inside of you. Your job is to find them and put them in place where they belong. It is no one else's job but your own. Other people may break you, but ultimately, you are responsible for your own healing and putting yourself back together. Not taking responsibility for it allows those who have hurt you to continue to do so. Healing yourself takes away their power over you. Meditate today knowing that you are already whole. You are complete. Remind yourself as much as you want to.

November 20

Got the munchies: pears

After dosing, get into your comfy spot and set a bowl of pear slices right by you. Be sure to use at least two varieties. This meditation is going to focus on your taste buds and other sensations. Keep your eyes closed so that you are not relying on your sense of sight. Use your sense of smell to take in the scent of each slice before you eat it. Can you identify the variety from the scent? Pay extreme attention to what you are doing as you take a bite. Feel your teeth sink into the pear. Experience the textures and flavor, singling them out as much as possible. Take your time and enjoy each of the slices, testing yourself to see if you can identify each one by the taste and scent. Use this type of meditation anytime you are eating for a fuller, richer connection with your food. Feel free to add music to this meditation or to substitute a different food item if you prefer.

November 21

Sadness

You do not have to suffer from seasonal affective disorder to experience sadness in the dark half of the year, but if you do, it does make this an even more challenging time than it already is. We experience grief deeply at the holidays, as it is a reminder our loved ones are no longer with us for special occasions. We grieve for them, time lost, innocence lost. We look back over the calendar year and grieve for our shortcomings and failures. Let yourself grieve. There is no dishonor in grief. It is okay to not feel as happy as you believe others around you to be. Some years are better than others, but grief must be lived through. You cannot go around it.

November 22
Strengthen yourself
Today is all about feeling strength.

Some people think being a bully makes them strong, but instead, bullying is a sign of weakness, with the perpetrator hiding their own insecurities.

Love, kindness, compassion, these are all qualities that can give us strength.

Meditate on what makes you feel strong. Are these positive qualities? Are they negative ones? What are your strengths and weaknesses?

November 23
Higher ideals
Start this meditation without the aid of cannabis. Instead, meditate on how you feel after each dose you take. Feel the THC as it takes you higher and higher with each dose until you finally hit your ideal high.

Reach out with your mind and feel yourself connect with the universe in oneness.

Relax and enjoy.

November 24
Comfort zone

Your comfort zone is your safe place. It's where you feel most at ease. Not necessarily a physical location, but one you can conjure in your mind when you need to.

Nothing threatening.

No worries.

Find your comfort zone in your mind, where you feel the safest. Know this is the place you can go to whenever you need a break or retreat from the chaos in the world around you.

Relax in your zone and enjoy.

November 25
Trance dance

As we dive deeper into the dark half of the year, we focus on our inner workings. We are multifaceted creatures who have many aspects to our inner workings and our makeup, both genetically and with our personalities. We are bits and pieces stuck together. Some of our pieces are big and take up a lot of room, time, and personality. But there are other pieces that are much smaller. We tend to overlook them, but all the same, they are a part of what makes us complete. For this trance dance, choose a song that represents one of the smaller aspects of you. I use "Rún" by SKÁLD as it celebrates a part of my heritage I wasn't in touch with growing up.

When you are ready, begin moving with the music. Block out everything but the sound of the music.

If physical limitations require it, remain seated while moving to the music.

You can "dance" with whatever body parts you want to use. Feel free to move in whatever way feels the most pleasing to you.

Allow the music to wash over and consume you.

Where does it take you?

November 26

Chant

"In the end,
we begin again.
Return, return, return.
Just as the new
will end again.
Return, return, return."

This chant reminds us of the cyclical pattern of life and nature. By the end of November, depending on where you live, the natural world looks dead. We must remind ourselves it is only at sleep and will return. New life will come again.

Repeat this chant throughout your meditation.

Try saying it in different intonations and at different speeds until you find your match.

How does this chant make you feel?

What does it mean to you?

November 27

Breathe it in: nutmeg oil

Nutmeg is an energizing scent. It is also used for drawing in luck, love, fidelity, and money.

Decide your purpose for working with the oil. Choose what correspondence(s) you want to focus on for this session. Since nutmeg is an energizing scent, you may want to use a sativa or sativa-dominant hybrid for this meditation (or perform it more than once comparing the difference between an indica and sativa strain.). Focus on what you would like to draw to you. If you focus on money, remember to focus on some luck to help draw it to you.

Prepare your meditation area ahead of time. You may want to use a diffuser to which you can add a few drops of oil. Use a self-lighting charcoal tablet in a fireproof container, and once the tablet is lit, add a few drops of oil to it for an intense burst of the scent. If you want to use the oil on your skin, be sure to add it to a carrier oil first. To keep it simple, sniff the oil from the bottle.

Use the oil in your chosen method. Close your eyes and inhale the scent deeply and slowly several times before allowing yourself to breathe normally again. Immerse yourself in the scent so that you feel its aura all around you. If you need to, take more slow, deep breaths to increase the intensity of the scent.

What feelings does this scent invoke in you? Does it bring back memories? Do you have a connection to this scent?

Feel free to add music to this meditation.

November 28
Smoke the herb: clove
Clove is very strong so only a little is needed. Clove is said to boost your memory, but it is also used for protection, courage, healing, and attracting money and love.

Combine your cannabis with some dried ground clove. I use a mix of about 90–95 percent cannabis to 5–10 percent herb, but you can adjust that according to your preferences.

When combining herbs with cannabis for the first time, always resort back to "slow and low." You are introducing a new combination of acids, proteins, and terpenes to your system. Give yourself time to see how it affects you, and that's all you have to do. Meditate on your reactions: How does it make you feel? Do you like it? How can you use this combination further in your practices?

November 29
Trust your feelings
Listen to your inner voice. The little voice inside your head that tells you right from wrong. Know your limits and trust your feelings. If you are not comfortable with a situation, there is a reason it is rubbing you the wrong way. How much confidence do you put into your feelings when they tell you something is off? Do you listen to your gut when it tries to warn you, or do you doubt your own intuition? How has that worked out for you?

November 30
Breathwork
Reflect over the past week, the past month, the past year. Think about the moments that have brought you the most peace, the most joy. Moments you know will remain some of your happiest memories down the road. As you reflect,

focus on your breathing and incorporate it into your memory. Deep breathing through memory recall allows you a deeper concentration to cement memories into place. The more senses involved in a memory, the easier it is for later recall. Feel free to add in soft music or aromatherapy scents.

✻ DECEMBER SHOPPING LIST ✻

Turquoise (December 10)

Dried crushed peppermint leaves (December 13)

Frankincense essential oil (December 19)

Oranges (December 27)

December 1
Solitude

Winter draws closer, the nights grow longer, and the need for solitude begins to arise. Following the cycle of life, now is the time to get ready for quiet introspection. How well do you do with solitude? Some people love it while others hate it. The more comfortable you are with yourself, the easier, and more welcome, solitude becomes. Do you enjoy it? Hate it? Have you had specific times when it scared you? Specific times you loved it? Meditate today on what solitude means for you.

December 2
Dormant

Like evergreens, we still show signs of life in the winter, but our energy goes dormant and turns inward. It is a time of outward rest. Visualize yourself as the spirit of any type of evergreen tree. Look around as the world around you changes colors, dries to brown, fades away, as you still stand tall and green. Inside, you feel warmth, wrapping your energy tight around you like a blanket to block out the cold. Focus on your inner core as the world fades away around you.

December 3
Inner wisdom

Listen to your inner wisdom. Let your high today bring forth whatever message your inner self has for you. The message you have been waiting for is here, ready for you now. Look into yourself to find the advice your inner wisdom wants you to know.

December 4
Integrity

Honesty, strong moral principles, being true to your word. These things require commitment, not a passing thought. It's hard work. Explore your commitment to your own integrity. What are your strongest principles? Do you find difficulty sometimes in sticking to them? What can you do to improve your integrity?

December 5
Perseverance

Reflect today on the perseverance your ancestors must have shown hundreds of years ago to survive through the winter and the dark half of the year—how they survived at any time of the year—but particularly through the winter months before electricity, before natural gas, before refrigeration. Visualize yourself living hundreds of years ago. See yourself living in the time of your ancestors past, enduring what they did.

December 6
Inspirational inklings

"For beautiful eyes, look for the good in others; for beautiful lips, speak only words of kindness; and for poise, walk with the knowledge that you are never alone."

—Audrey Hepburn[20]

Audrey tells us it us up to us to see the good in others and to be the example we want to see in the world. Some days, this is more difficult than others. Some days, we feel that the world and its negativity is getting to us and that we are alone in our struggle to do the right thing. Remind yourself, we are here only for a short while. How others affect us is entirely up to us. We can look for the negativity, or we can look for the positivity. Even at the worst, know you are never alone.

---

20. Maggie Parker, "13 of Audrey Hepburn's Most Inspiring Quotes," Time, May 4, 2016, https://time.com/4316700/audrey-hepburn-inspiring-quotes/.

Reflect on these words from Audrey Hepburn. How can you incorporate this wisdom into your life?

December 7
Intuition

Intuition is a powerful tool once you learn how to use it. Let your intuition guide you in your meditation today. Where does your intuition need to direct your focus? Follow its lead to receive a needed message.

December 8
Migration

Birds travel every year from the northern parts of the hemisphere to southern areas as a part of their migration path. They know to leave the area that has become too harsh for their safe survival. They know to leave an area that has made their survival difficult and to move to a place of warmth and abundance to meet their needs. They move on when things are too difficult for survival and come back when life and abundance has returned to the land.

We can learn from the pattern of birds and leave those situations that have become unsafe or too difficult to survive in. Meditate today contemplating if there are aspects of your life that need to be left behind in order for you to thrive.

December 9

Call of the wild: whale song

Do an online search for "whale song."

Find a clip that is a good length for your meditation time or use a repeat feature.

Play the song and meditate on it as you listen.

Do you like this sound? Dislike the sound?

Let the sound encompass you.

How does it make you feel?

December 10

Get stoned: turquoise

Turquoise is a blue/green stone that resonates with friendship, courage, happiness, luck, emotional balance, astral travel, communication, protection, and prosperity.

Turquoise is a very versatile stone and can be used to assist you in many ways. Which of these needs could turquoise help you fulfill? How can you combine qualities together to create a unique, personalized stone for you? It's very well rounded so there are many possibilities—think about being new to a job, school, even a town. Looking to meet new people? Friendship, courage, happiness, luck, emotional balance, communication, protection, and prosperity could all give that a boost.

Get into your comfy spot and hold the stone in your hand out in front of you.

Examine the stone with your eyes and your fingers.
Feel the stone as you hold it tightly in your hand.
Hold the stone close to your heart.
Meditate on the stone and how it feels to you.
Carry this stone with you whenever you feel the need.

December 11
Selfless service

We are reminded throughout the holidays how many people throughout our local community, our country, and the rest of the world are in need. Countless organizations exist to help people, or other beneficiaries, and these organizations rely heavily on the talents, skills, and time of people just like you who volunteer. Meditate today on what selfless service you can give, not just at the holidays but year-round. The need for volunteers is constant; make a commitment to get started.

December 12
Peaceful Rest

Let today's meditation be about peaceful rest. Allow any negativities to slip from your mind. No worries. No stress. Just restful peace and quiet. Go to your sacred place to rest and rejuvenate. Come back cleansed and fully recharged.

December 13
Smoke the herb: peppermint

Peppermint is a plant of energy. It makes you feel energized, mentally stimulated, more psychically aware, possibly even a bit lustful. It gives and builds energy in different aspects.

Combine your cannabis with some dried ground peppermint. Use a mix of about 70 percent cannabis to 30 percent herb, but you can adjust that according to your preferences.

When combining herbs with cannabis for the first time, always resort back to "slow and low." You are introducing a new combination of acids, proteins, and terpenes to your system. Give yourself time to see how it affects you, and that's all you have to do. Meditate on your reactions: How does it make you feel? Do you like it? How can you use this combination further in your practices?

December 14
Chill lounge

Embrace the darkness. Embrace the rest it brings to us— the chance to recharge. Turn your focus and workings inward. The outer world is at rest, at peace. Time slows for a while. Solitude. Reflection. Contemplation.

Find a song that reflects this aspect of nature for you, one that helps you embrace the workings of the dark.

I enjoy "And Winter Came" by Enya.

Play your music while you are in your comfy spot. Let not only the music but any lyrics flow over you, and listen deeply and intently. Where does the music take you? How does it make you feel?

December 15
Stillness

Life is hectic. Allow yourself to relax in a moment of stillness. No worries, no plans, no stress, no deadlines. It is only you in your moment. The world can do without you while you soak in the beauty of stillness.

December 16
A blessed idea

We are all responsible for making our world a kinder, more loving, gentler place. Meditate today on how you can contribute to this goal. What actions, what ideas can you conceive and implement to bless others in the world around you? What need in others can you help fulfill?

December 17
Forgive yourself

Forgiving yourself can be one of the hardest things to do. We often hold ourselves to a higher standard than we do others. Some people hold themselves to lower standards as well.

Either way, forgiving oneself can be extremely difficult, while also being emotionally healthy. Heartfelt forgiveness of oneself helps build empathy for others. Whether you are forgiven by other people or not is out of your control, but you are in control when it comes to forgiving yourself.

Meditate on what you need to forgive yourself for. What does forgiveness look like to you? How will forgiveness change you?

Allow yourself the chance to grieve, if necessary. Know that forgiving yourself is an act of compassionate self-love.

December 18
Pettiness
Pettiness simply isn't pretty. It's irritating, annoying, childish, and yet so many of us do it all the time. Use today's meditation to think about the little things that annoy you. The little things that you could let slip by, but you don't. How do you differentiate between what is a big annoyance and what is a small one? What does your own pettiness say about you?

December 19
Breathe it in: frankincense oil

Frankincense is a very spiritual oil. It is used during meditations throughout the world and in rituals from a variety of religions. Frankincense is also used for protection, banishing negative entities, and consecration.

Decide your purpose for working with the oil. Choose what correspondence(s) you want to focus on for this session. This is a wonderful oil for spiritual meditations for connecting with the divine or your higher self, or it can be used for an aura cleanse.

Prepare your meditation area ahead of time. You may want to use a diffuser to which you can add a few drops of oil. Use a self-lighting charcoal tablet in a fireproof container, and once the tablet is lit, add a few drops of oil to it for an intense burst of the scent. If you want to use the oil on your skin, be sure to add it to a carrier oil first. To keep it simple, sniff the oil from the bottle.

Use the oil in your chosen method. Close your eyes and inhale the scent deeply and slowly several times before allowing yourself to breathe normally again. Immerse yourself in the scent so that you feel its aura all around you. If you need to, take more slow, deep breaths to increase the intensity of the scent.

What feelings does this scent invoke in you? Does it bring back memories? Do you have a connection to this scent?

Feel free to add music to this meditation.

December 20

Chant

"The nights are long
the air is cold;
the sun will return
with strength so bold."

Winter is here. It is important to remember this is a time of rest in anticipation of the light to come. It is a temporary break. While you can take shelter in rest, know that the cycle continues and someday, once again, the time for rest will be over and the time for action will begin. Allow yourself to connect with this cycle of nature.

Repeat this chant throughout your meditation.

Try saying it in different intonations and at different speeds until you find your match.

How does this chant make you feel?

What does it mean to you?

December 21
Make an offering
Give up an offering to either your deities, your guides, the universe, or your community.

Physical offerings can range from an outdoor winter feast prepared on an old table for the wildlife to enjoy to tying scarves around poles and trees in areas frequented by homeless people.

Mead, oranges, and pomegranates all make appropriate offerings to deities.

Serving in a soup kitchen, homeless shelter, or wrapping and delivering gifts for charities are all popular volunteer opportunities at this time of year.

Choose an offering that comes from your heart.

December 22
A light in the darkness
The promise winter gives us is a light in the darkness. Through the darkest nights, the days begin growing longer, even as the cold remains. It is a sign to us that warmth will follow, and the world will one day reawaken in all its natural beauty.

Connect with the light in the darkness in your meditation. Warmth surrounded by coldness. Feel the promise of the hope it holds within.

December 23

Embrace the darkness

Perform this meditation in the darkest spot you can. A windowless room with no lights on would be the most ideal location.

We are taught the dark is evil. Bad.

This is not, never has been, and never will be true.

Dark is the counterpart to light. It is light's other half to make the whole.

Dark gives us quiet and rest.

Spend this meditation in the dark, but don't just sit there and try to figure out if you can see things. Close your eyes and see if you can feel things—not with your hands, but psychically. Can you send your spirit, your aura, into the room to feel where things are?

Feel comfort in the dark and connect with it.

December 24

The animals speak

There is an old tale that claims at midnight on Christmas Eve the animals are blessed with the ability to speak. Have fun in your meditation tonight. Meet with the animal spirits of your choice; ask them to come to visit with you and to tell you their tales.

December 25
The holiday season

No matter what holidays you choose to celebrate, or you may choose none at all, allow today to be a day of rest and recuperation in your meditation. Head into your sacred space for comfort and peace. Surround yourself with love, joy, appreciation. No other worries, no other stress. Only peace.

December 26
Feel the shift

Winter has officially arrived; the holidays are quickly passing by. The darkness, the solitude, the time for seasonal rest is here. Our thoughts can shift from the outer world and happenings to our inner self, to the work we need to do internally over these dark days.

Meditate today on the work to come. You are at rest now, but know in the coming days, inner work must be done to allow you to heal and grow. Feel the shift as you move from the outer world to the inner.

December 27
Got the munchies: oranges

After dosing, get into your comfy spot and set a bowl of orange slices right by you. This meditation is going to focus on your taste buds and other sensations. Keep your eyes closed so that you are not relying on your sense of sight. Use your sense of smell to take in the scent of each slice before you eat it. Pay extreme attention to what you are doing as you take a bite. Feel your teeth sink into the orange. Experience the textures and flavor, singling them out as much as possible. Take your time and enjoy the orange. Use this type of meditation anytime you are eating for a fuller, richer connection with your food.

December 28
Closure
The end of the calendar year is close by. Take time today to give yourself closure where needed. What can you say goodbye to and leave in the old year? What no longer serves you? Cut ties that bind you down instead of holding you up. Endings lead to new beginnings.

December 29
Trance dance
From children believing in flying reindeer to the enchantment of nature as billions and billions of snowflakes, each an individual work of art, fall from the sky, winter has its own magic. The calendar is almost at an end, and there is anticipation and hope for the new year in the air.

Choose a song that celebrates the magic of winter. Whether it is a slow or fast song is up to you, whichever you feel works best for you at this time.

I use "Wizards in Winter" by Trans-Siberian Orchestra.

When you are ready, begin moving with the music. Block out everything but the sound of the music.

If physical limitations require it, remain seated while moving to the music.

You can "dance" with whatever body parts you want to use. Feel free to move in whatever way feels the most pleasing to you.

Allow the music to wash over and consume you.

Where does it take you?

December 30
Breathwork

Let's end the month, and the year, with some good releasing breathwork. Anything that has been weighing you down, anything that has been holding you back, let it go. Just. Let. It. Go. With a big swoooooooooooooosh. Problems at work? Let them go. Issues at home? Let them go. Every negative thought, iota, speck. Let. It. All. Go. Each breath deeper than the next. Reach down in, and pull out whatever is left that needs to get out and let it go. For right now, for this moment in time, let it all go. Let each breath cleanse you until it is all gone. Release.

December 31
The end of a year

The end of a year brings hope for the next one to be better. Do not focus on the bad events from the past year. Learn from mistakes, but today, spend your meditation in celebration of fun, accomplishments, and happy remembrances. Look forward to the new year with hopeful anticipation.

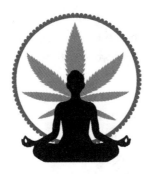

Chapter 2
Lunar Meditations

When performing a new or full moon meditation, you will want to focus on the correspondences not only for the moon phase but for the month as well.

Full moons correspond with working on bringing positives into your life, creativity, physical energy, completing and perfecting your ideas, projects, plans, and possibly an increase in your psychic energy.

New moons correspond with banishing things from your life (such as bad habits), healing, resting, and possibly an increase in your psychic energy.

Each month also corresponds to a theme, which will be reflected in each of the moon meditations.

Lunar meditations work with the moon and feminine energies.

January Full Moon

The January full moon, also known as the Wolf Moon or Snow Moon, is the right time to start new positive, creative, or physical projects. While the new moon focuses on a new beginning through the end of negativity, the full moon focuses on new beginnings by drawing in more positivity.

Meditate on what new positivity you can bring into your life. If there is something you have wanted to try, do it! Visualize your new project, habit, plan—whatever it is—happening and turning out how you want. Visualize a successful outcome. Feel the joy it brings to you. Your meditation is a practice run to show the impact your new beginning can make.

January New Moon

January is all about beginnings. It's the beginning of the new year and, traditionally, people see it as a fresh start. People set goals and make resolutions to work on the rest of the year.

When you add the moon phase into the mix, the new moon is good for getting rid of things, along with healing and resting.

This combination makes the January new moon the ideal time to work on banishing unhealthy habits from your life.

Meditate on what unhealthy habits you need to banish. Remember—cannabis allows you to see yourself clearer when you let it. Let cannabis open your eyes to see what unhealthy habits you can eliminate.

February Full Moon

The February full moon, also known as the Snow Moon, Storm Moon, or Hunger Moon, is ideal for working through challenges in a positive manner. Use your meditation to brainstorm creative and positive solutions to the challenges you are facing. Now is the ideal time to think outside of the box to solve stubborn problems.

In addition, the February full moon is ideal for rededicating yourself to projects, goals, resolutions, whatever area in your life needs reaffirmation of your dedication. Give yourself a status check of the things you are working to accomplish, both short-term and long-term goals. You can meditate through this as a second meditation if you choose.

February New Moon

February is for dealing with challenges, and for purifying and dedicating oneself. At the new moon, meditate on eliminating challenges and other negativities from your life. The new moon corresponds to banishment, so these are challenges you want to get rid of; they are not the ones you need to work through and overcome for a better life. They are the annoying little things that you allow to distract you that you don't have to. These things can disappear without any negative consequences. Meditate on what these things are for you, let the universe guide you into eliminating those aspects. Getting rid of these negativities is another step in healing your life and spirit.

March Full Moon

While the new moon helps to get rid of blockages and obstacles in the way of hope or success, the full moon helps build creativity and plans to ensure our hopes can be fulfilled and success is within grasp.

Also known as the Worm Moon, Seed Moon, Plow Moon, or Moon of Winds, the names for this month's moon celebrate the idea of hope and success. The worms have been successful in surviving the winter and come out of the ground to announce spring is here. The names Seed and Plow Moon reflect the preparing of land for crops for a successful harvest. These events sing of successful survival and hope for the new year and harvest.

Meditate on your own plowing and choosing of seeds for your own hopeful success. Use the creativity from the moon and cannabis to plan out how the crop of your success should be cultivated for the best results.

March New Moon

March brings with it hope and the joy of success. In ancient times to as recent as a hundred years ago, surviving until spring was a great accomplishment. While technology has increased the chances of not freezing or starving to death, we still associate success with March. After the cold and dark of winter, there is the time of rebirth. But rebirth takes just that—time. Now is not the time to give up. There are bigger and better successes in store for you.

At the new moon, we want to banish the things that interfere with our hope and success. What in your life brings negativity and attempts to cut down on your hope or success? Meditate on if you have these issues (whether it's caused by yourself or other people) and, if so, how you can eliminate them.

April Full Moon

The April moon is full, and it is time to draw the things to us that we want in our lives. Known as the Pink Moon or Seed Moon, use it to get your "seeds" planted, watered, and on their way to growth and abundance. In this meditation, see the start of your goals, the first steps you need to take toward them being completed. Visualize yourself successfully doing what needs to be done, step-by-step, to cultivate your plans into a successful "harvest." Draw that which you need to you. Whatever your plans and goals are, now is the time to implement them.

April New Moon

Use the new moon to pick out any "weeds" you need to from your garden of life. Are there things in your life that are going to interfere in the planting and growth of your seeds? These are your weeds, and you need to keep them under control so they do not choke out what you want to accomplish.

Meditate on your "garden." What weeds do you see that you will have to deal with? Remember that when we do not remove a weed by the root, it can often grow back. How much weeding you want to do is up to you, but remember your main goal is to make your dreams grow and thrive. People should keep their weeds out of your garden and worry about cultivating their own dreams to thrive. Weed out any negatives.

May Full Moon

The May full moon corresponds with good health, wisdom, love, and romance.

What else could anyone else want all rolled up into one! The May full moon is bursting with magic. Known as the Flower Moon, Hare Moon, or Merry Moon, the May moon is for drawing in all the above qualities in abundance. It is a very fertile time! Visualize what you want to draw into your life in any of these categories. Remember there is a difference between love and romance, so this can pertain to any type of love—love of your family, your friends, or even a pet. Are any of these areas lacking in your life? Meditate on how you can change that.

May New Moon

Once May rolls along, we are ready for a little break from our main focus of the year. While we continue to tend to our plans and goals, we can turn our focus to other areas in our lives. May is the time for working on health, love, romance, and wisdom. At the new moon, we need to rid ourselves of the things that interfere in these aspects of our lives.

Is there a habit you have that is affecting your health? Now is the time to meditate on ending the habit.

Are you in a relationship that is not bringing you the love you need? Now is the time to meditate on either ending the relationship or ending negative issues within the relationship.

Gaining wisdom doesn't mean furthering your education—it means learning from your mistakes. Have you consistently made the same mistake, and therefore, are not gaining wisdom from it? Now is the time to meditate on eliminating the same detrimental course of action.

Remember, at the new moon, we need to rid ourselves of obstacles in the way. At the full moon, we draw desired energies toward us.

June Full Moon

Strawberry Moon, Lover's Moon, Mead Moon, Honey Moon, Rose Moon.

With names like these, it is no wonder the June full moon corresponds with sensuality, romance, and sex. Many weddings take place in June as it is a time for lovers.

A late-night outdoor meditation focusing on drawing these intentions to you could be quite sensual. Remember, there is a difference between feeling sensual and being sexual; however, cannabis does heighten both experiences. Having your partner join you for a joint meditation focusing on your connection to one another could be quite romantic and intimate. Use this meditation however it serves you best.

June New Moon

If life were only about love and romance, it would be so much easier. But it is not. There is work, kids, bills, stress, aches and pains, medical issues, too much to do, too little time, and some things get pushed to the wayside. You may not feel romantic; maybe you have a low libido. If you want to change those things, then now is the time to work on removing these blockages from your life. If you are happily single, are there any obstacles that need to be worked on in other loving-type relationships in your life?

Use the power of the new moon to deal with those obstacles. Meditate on solutions to eliminate whatever issues you are having.

July Full Moon

The July full moon is at the height of summer—the time when the sun is at its full strength. Both of these major influences are at the peak of their power, and this lends strength to your own, to your success, and to your health. Meditating on plans for success helps bring them into reality.

The July full moon is also known to be a time of enchantment when fairy folk abound in areas rich in flora and fauna. If you perform a meditation in their space, be sure to leave behind an offering.

This full moon goes by the names Buck Moon, Hay Moon, Wort Moon, or Thunder Moon.

July New Moon

What is standing in your way of success? Do you sabotage yourself? Do you have difficulties blowing your own horn? Are you a procrastinator? Whatever it is, the July new moon is perfect for ridding it from your life.

Meditate on what obstacles you need to eliminate that get in the way of your health, your success, or your personal strength. Visualize how these changes will affect you and improve your life. Seeing yourself strong and successful is the first step to achieving strength and success. Build yourself stairs to get over the obstacles you can't seem to tear down. Sometimes we need to go around or over instead of plowing straight through. Where does your path need to take you?

August Full Moon

The harvests are beginning, and the August full moon represents this abundance. The seasonal energies tell you to keep doing the things that are working for you and giving you a good response. If there are areas that aren't doing so well, it's time to decide if you want to try a new approach or focus your energies elsewhere.

Evaluate your harvest. What is working well for you? What do you need to revisit with new ideas?

The August full moon is known by several names including Sturgeon Moon, Corn Moon, and Barley Moon —all relating to their abundance.

August New Moon

During the August full moon, you evaluate what is working for you and creating abundance in your life. At the new moon, you need to evaluate what is not working for you and make decisions about how to eliminate those instances from your life. What makes you weak or nonproductive? Have you tried something that everyone says works for them but it doesn't work for you? There is a saying that the definition of insanity is doing the same thing over and over and expecting different results—well, we are all a bit insane! We do this to ourselves a lot. We do things out of habit or because it is referred to us, but it doesn't really *work*.

Take the time to really look at what does not work for you. Get it out of your life. Let it go. Visualize yourself getting rid of what you need to and investigate your new possible future outcomes.

September Full Moon

The energy of the September full moon is very similar to the August full moon with a focus on abundance and prosperity. Protection also comes into play as a hint of the darkness to come during the long days of winter.

Known by names such as Corn Moon, Harvest Moon, Wine Moon, and Singing Moon, it is easy to see abundance is forefront.

Your meditation should look to preparing for your future. What positive steps do you need to take to ensure protection and stability through the next season?

September New Moon

As you plan for your future security, it is also necessary to perceive and eliminate any threats to said security. What may be standing in your way of a secure future? What obstacles are in your way that must be removed to ensure continued abundance and security? Do you hold yourself back? Do you have health conditions that must be monitored continually? Do you work in a field being downsized? Look at where your weaknesses lie.

Remember, sometimes subtraction gives us a greater win than addition. Less truly can be more.

October Full Moon

The October full moon is highly associated with death, endings, and new beginnings. Blood Moon, Harvest Moon, and Hunter's Moon all predict a final outcome for some, while ensuring survival for others. With the last harvest being done in October, the slaughter of animals, and the last chance to hunt before winter, it's easy to see where these names came from.

Death can be mourned as a life is celebrated. Endings can be painful and joyful at the same time. New beginnings bring mystery and adventure.

Psychic energy is high and spiritual contacts are made easily. Reach out to loved ones beyond the veil for connection with them, or into the universe for connection with your higher self.

Meditations done at the October full moon can focus on any of these aspects.

October New Moon

At the new moon, we remember that new life comes after death, but first a time of rest is needed. We remember it is a time of sacrifice so that others may live. It is a time to honor the shadow side. We do not fear the dark. The dark is not bad or evil. It is only dark. We are at peace and our energies shift, downgrade. We slow to a repose.

October lunar meditations are deeply moving as the energies at this time of year are highly spiritual in nature due to the thinned veil. This thinning allows for easy contact with all other spiritual beings, including our higher selves.

November Full Moon

The November full moon, with names such as Beaver Moon, Snow Moon, Dark Moon, Fog Moon, Mad Moon, or Mourning Moon (if it is the last full moon before the winter solstice), draws family and friends together. The psychic energies are also ripe for divination.

You can perform a full moon meditation focusing on bringing family and friends together in peace, or you could turn your attentions to a more spiritual meditation.

A free form meditation taking note of what comes to you can easily be used for divinatory purposes by analyzing the symbols present in your meditation.

November New Moon

While the full moon brings family and friends together, the new moon may bring up issues that need to be dealt with instead of being left to simmer or moved to the back burner. The new moon is ideal for healing, so mending grievances now goes a long way. During holidays, things can get hectic and stressful. Many families do not do well being in close proximity with one another; even families that love each other greatly find themselves stressed out and bothered more easily. You may have issues yourself you do not want to deal with; now is not the time to set them aside.

Meditate on ways you can bring healing into needed situations.

December Full Moon

Known as the Cold Moon, Wolf Moon, Oak Moon, and Moon of Long Nights, the December full moon corresponds to building hope and attracting healing. Hope was very important to have during the long, cold winter nights. The full moon was a beacon of this hope and still serves as a symbol of hope today.

Now is the time for rest and healing. It is time for a break before we begin turning our energy inward during the winter months. Let your meditation today focus on the hopes you have this Cold Moon.

December New Moon

The new moon of December is when we get rid of any negativities interfering with our hope or healing. Is something standing in your way or giving you doubt? Doubt negates hope. Meditate on any obstacles, negativities, or doubts you have regarding your own healing or hope.

Do you have something holding you back from moving forward? The hardest negativity to overcome is also the most important one—denial. Until an issue or problem is recognized and defined, it has no hope of being solved. Look for any negativity that is holding you back. Now is an ideal time to face it.

Blue Moon

The original meaning of a blue moon was the third full moon in a season that contained four full moons. This was called a seasonal blue moon. The term shifted to include a second full moon within a calendar month. With either definition, a blue moon is rare, happening every few years.

Astrologically, a blue moon will have different correspondences depending on which zodiac sign it is passing through, so we will work with the calendrical correspondences.

A blue moon is the perfect time to recount, celebrate, and appreciate your grandest accomplishments. The processes you undertook for these achievements have shaped you into who you are.

Meditate on your accomplishments and what they say about you.

Black Moon

A black moon is a similar concept to a blue moon, but instead of referring to a full moon, it describes the second new moon in a calendar month. Black moons have a seasonal version which occur every thirty-two months.

This is a time to let deep, dark emotional issues come to the surface in your meditation. It is time for your subconscious to reveal its hidden secrets. While painful, this is how we heal. Lower your walls and inhibitions to see objectively what you need to see.

Lunar Eclipse

A lunar eclipse can drain your energy and make you more emotional at the same time. Emotional healing done during a lunar eclipse is very powerful as it allows you to go inside on a deeper level to confront what hidden issues you must. Combined with the objectivity gifted by THC, be prepared for a possible emotional overload as you work through opening yourself up and looking inside during this meditation.

The lunar eclipse guides you on your soul path and shows you the next steps of your journey. Open your heart and mind to the messages given as you look deep inside.

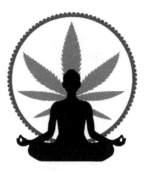

Chapter 3
Solar Meditations

Solar meditations work with the sun and masculine energies. They include the equinoxes, solstices, eclipses, and the annual solar event of your birthday.

Vernal Equinox

The vernal, or spring, equinox is all about balance. Night and day are in equal amounts. After today, the days will continue to grow longer and the nights shorter until the summer solstice. Spend your meditation visualizing yourself in perfect balance. You may want to visualize this in the literal physical sense (perhaps see yourself standing in a tall, balanced tree pose), or in a more figurative aspect such as weighing areas of your life on a scale to ensure all is in proper balance. Whichever works for you, the balance is the key.

Summer Solstice

The longest day and shortest night of the year comprises the summer solstice. It symbolizes prosperity and abundance. Let your meditation focus on your own prosperity and abundance. Be sure to offer up thanks to the universe for the blessings you have been bestowed.

Autumnal Equinox

Once again, we find the light and dark in equal balance. This time around though, the power of the sun is weakening. Days are growing shorter and, after today, the nights obtain dominance. Prepare for the shift of thoughts and workings turning inward as the dark half of the year begins.

The energy shifts from growth to harvesting. Stabilization soon to be followed by decline. The winding down of the year has begun. Some people feel the energy shift as strongly as the first slow down at the end of the roller coaster ride. The brakes are being gently applied.

Center yourself today to ground and prepare for the change to come.

Winter Solstice

The winter solstice is the longest night of the year. Making it through the dark nights with the promise of the sun's return as days begin to grow longer was a granting of the gift of life.

The winter solstice reflects overcoming our greatest obstacles, our biggest challenges, or our most harrowing fears.

Reflect today on what you have overcome. Let go of grief and hold on to the promise of the return of the light.

Solar Eclipse

The solar eclipse ushers in changes from external forces outside of us. While these changes are generally positive, they are often unexpected changes to the path we were on. Meditate today with the power of the solar eclipse to reveal a new direction for you to take.

Birthday

It is your day, allow your meditation to be a gift to yourself. Whatever you need from your meditation today, whether it be a celebration of your life, a recognition of gained wisdom, or a precious moment alone, gift yourself according to what you need.

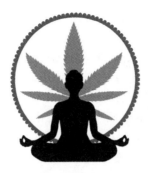

Chapter 4
Sabbat Meditations

The eight sabbats are celebrated by a variety of Pagan traditions and those who live closely with the earth. Each one having a different focus, they combine together to create the Wheel of the Year. No matter what your spiritual beliefs are, the Wheel of the Year follows seasonal patterns and is ripe with reasons to celebrate and meditate.

Imbolc

Imbolc is celebrated about halfway between Yule and Ostara. It is the traditional mark of the beginning of spring. The grounds are beginning to thaw. The lakes resume showing off their ebb and flow of the tidal pulls. In the spiritual aspect, the goddess—Mother Earth—begins to wake from her winter slumber. It is time to begin the mental preparations for that which you want to plant and harvest in your life over the coming seasons.

With thoughts turned inward during the dark half of the year, you have had time to focus on where your next work needs to be done. Use your Imbolc meditation to explore what you want to plant in your garden of life. Follow the energies of nature and begin to awaken yourself from your long winter nap.

Ostara

Celebrated at the vernal equinox as the first official day of spring, the theme of Ostara is one of renewal and rebirth. The goddess is young, playful, and fertile. We rejoice in the reawakening of the earth. Life begins anew.

We begin tilling our life garden. We prepare to begin working on the goals we created at Imbolc—the seeds we wish to plant. We know what we want, now we must plan how to get it.

Meditate on what your next steps for your goals should be.

Beltane

Beltane is a Pagan fertility festival. The goddess in the form of the maiden mates with the god.

It is when we ask for blessings upon our seeds and soil and the planting takes place. We begin watering, fertilizing, and providing sunlight to ensure maximum growth.

The first steps of our goals are taken. Our plans are set in motion, and we take steps to nourish them toward completion. Meditate on your next steps.

Midsummer

Midsummer takes place at the summer solstice, which is the official start of the astronomical summer season. The sun is at its height of power in the Northern Hemisphere, and the longest day is at hand.

The goddess grows a child inside her as her god protects her and his land.

The sun's strength reminds us of our strength and promises hard work will be rewarded. We continue to nourish our projects and goals so they will flourish and soon reach their completion and harvest.

Meditate and evaluate the growth of your garden. What are your next steps?

Lughnasadh

Lughnasadh is the first of the three harvests. The goddess grows more abundant in her pregnancy as life flourishes all around her. We celebrate the strength of the sun god and the abundance he provides.

Some goals, smaller, shorter projects, should be finishing up now as we begin to bring in the first fruits of the harvest and begin to enjoy the rewards from our labor. As these earliest goals mature, energy and resources can be diverted to more complicated, long-term goals.

Meditate on what you are able to harvest. What resources can you divert elsewhere?

Mabon

The second of the three harvests and celebrated at the autumnal equinox. It is the spiritual celebration in which we give thanks for all that we have. The god and goddess have given us a plentiful bounty, and we rejoice in thankfulness. The God sacrifices himself to ensure the survival of his people. (Different traditions honor this sacrifice at different times.)

The bulk of your goals should be in midlife stages. Your plans and projects are fruitful and provide you with sustenance and a sense of accomplishment. Your successes encourage you.

With the day and night equal, you are reminded the growing season will soon come to an end and fields will go fallow once again.

Meditate on what you have accomplished so far. Visualize the rest of your successful harvest.

Samhain

The third and final harvest. The world around us has gone fallow. The last of the crops have been brought in and the herds culled of the weak and sick. The goddess mourns her lost love.

We wrap up our plans for the year and re-evaluate where we stand. Some goals we may continue to work on while others are cut or set aside for storage to be revisited later. Resources may be limited during the dark half of the year. Time and money are shifted to different priorities as holidays and families take precedence.

The year is at an end and the time for rest is here.

Evaluate where you stand with your projects and goals and prepare yourself for rest.

Yule

The winter solstice, the shortest day and longest night of the year. It is the rebirth of the sun as the days will now begin to grow stronger in their fight against the night. The son is also reborn as the goddess gives birth once again to the god.

We enjoy this time of rest. We bring together those we love and cherish and celebrate accomplishments from throughout the year. We are in a peaceful hibernation—a time between death and rebirth. We wait for the coming light and recuperate our strength.

Enjoy your time of rest. Your work, for now, is done.

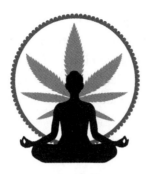

Chapter 5
Elemental Meditations

Elemental meditations correspond to the five elements of air, fire, water, earth, and spirit.

Air

The element air is associated with the direction east. It is concerned with new ideas and beginnings. It rules communication, intellect, and social relationships.

Face east when performing your air meditation either outdoors or near an open window or running fan.

Visualize yourself floating, on a cloud, in a sacred space, or in whatever way says "air" to you. Feel breezes and winds of energy as they blow through and around you. Air cleanses you and opens you up to communication, love, friendship, and joy.

Use lavender, violet, or rosemary incense or oil to add to your air-based meditation. You may also hold a yellow stone.

Fire

Fire is associated with the direction south. It focuses on energy, courageousness, passion, assertiveness, stimulation, and creativity.

Focus on fire when you need a boost in any of the above qualities.

Visualize or perform your meditation near a small campfire or light a candle. The flames of the fire are charged with energy to fuel your passion, your creativity, your courage. Take what you need from the energy of the fire.

Use lime, orange, lemongrass, or neroli scents to add to your fire-based meditation. You may also hold on to a red stone.

Water

Water is associated with the direction of west. It centers on emotion, sensitivity, intuition, and romance. Anytime you need to boost or calm these aspects, perform a water-themed meditation. Performing this meditation near or in water (such as is in a bath or hot tub) adds to the energy.

Face west while floating in water or visualizing yourself in it. Water washes over you, cleansing, calming, reenergizing the aspects you wish. Waves and currents of energy flow around and through you.

Use lemon, lily of the valley, or lotus scents to enhance your water meditation. Additionally, hold a blue stone or add blue stones to the water you soak in.

Earth

Earth is associated with the direction north. It centers on the practical, the skillful. It is grounded and literally "down to earth."

Focus on earth and its energy when you need to ground yourself. Let it pull scattered energies into a better alignment.

While facing north, visualize yourself sitting on a forest floor, thick with rich vegetation. (Or perform your meditation in a similar location.) Feel the energy of the earth as it reaches out, looping rooted tendrils around you, gently binding you to the ground.

Use pine, cedar, sage, vetiver, or cypress scents to add to your earth-based meditation or hold on to a green stone.

Spirit

Spirit is the prime elemental in all living things; it is intangible yet binds the other elements together to make us whole. It is through spirit we are connected to all things and to the universe.

Meditate on the element of spirit. Connect to the oneness of the universe and visualize spirit within you. Feel spirit within you. Reach out to the oneness and feel for other connections to spirit. Connect with spirit and enjoy.

Spirit is associated with purple or a clear white light energy. Amethyst and quartz are excellent for spirit work. Use frankincense, myrrh, or patchouli when working with spirit.

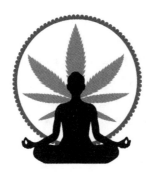

Chapter 6
Aura and Chakra Meditations

The meditations in this section can be used in place of any other daily meditation or in addition. These meditations are to help you focus your attention on cleansing your aura and chakras. You may want to set up a practice where you cleanse your aura and chakras once a month. You can either do them all in the same day or choose one for each day of the week.

Aura Cleanse

Negativity bogs us down. It clouds our aura and doesn't allow us to reflect our true light. To cleanse your aura, get into your comfy spot after medicating and visualize a cleansing, bright white light circling over your head. The light continues spinning in circles as it lowers closer and closer to the top of your head. As it reaches just above your hair, the white light begins swirling larger and larger. It reaches past your shoulders, growing enough to encompass your entire body as it slowly moves downward while consistently spinning and swirling around and through you. Visualize this bright light cleansing and purifying your aura, removing negativities, removing cloudiness. The white light leaves your aura bright, shining, and energized.

Root Chakra (Muladhara)

When the root chakra, located at the base of your spine, is out of balance or blocked, you may experience fear and anxiety. An out of balance root chakra results in excessive negativity and insecurity. It makes you feel under attack and results in greed and can even trigger eating disorders. Your root chakra is associated with earth; it is what keeps you feeling grounded and stable. When it is blocked, you are thrown off your game.

Cleanse your root chakra by visualizing streaks of white light, lightning, absorbing into your body through your outer appendages—your fingertips, your tippy toes, the crown chakra just at the top of your head. It penetrates your body, following ley lines to reach your root chakra at the base of your spine. The white light flows into the chakra and begins spiraling, cleansing, rebalancing as it goes. Suddenly the white light changes into a bright, blood red. The spiraling increases as energy radiates like a firework exploding in the night sky. The spiraling gently slows to a comfortable pulse, still shining bright. You are balanced and cleansed.

Sacral Chakra (Swadhisthana)

The sacral chakra is located in your lower belly and is associated with the element of water. It rules over your emotions, relationships, sexuality, and creativity. When your sacral chakra is out of balance or blocked, you may experience dependencies or addictions, out of control emotions or the opposite—no emotions at all. You may have difficulty establishing fantasy from reality.

Cleanse your sacral chakra by visualizing streaks of white light shooting into your body through your outer appendages—your fingertips, your tippy toes, the crown chakra just at the top of your head. It penetrates your body, following ley lines to reach your sacral chakra in the middle of your lower belly. The white light flows into the chakra and begins spiraling, cleansing, rebalancing as it goes. The white light changes into a strong, bold orange. The spiraling increases as energy radiates outward, cleansing until pure. The spiraling gently slows to a comfortable pulse, still shining bright. You are balanced and cleansed.

Solar Plexus Chakra (Manipura)

Located in the upper belly area, the solar plexus chakra is associated with fire. It rules over your personal power, will power, intellect, taking control over your life, and decision making. When it is blocked or out of balance, you may act like an overbearing tyrant, or the opposite—too helpless to make the simplest decisions. Imbalances cause you to be manipulative and to abuse your power. You may make poor decisions with little to no thought put into them.

Cleanse your solar plexus chakra by visualizing streaks of white light absorbing into your body through your outer appendages—your fingertips, your tippy toes, the crown chakra just at the top of your head. It penetrates your body, following ley lines to reach your solar plexus chakra in your upper belly region. The white light flows into the chakra and begins spiraling, cleansing, rebalancing as it goes. The white light changes into a brilliant yellow. The spiraling increases as energy radiates like rays from the sun. The spiraling gently slows to a comfortable pulse, still shining bright. You are balanced and cleansed.

Heart Chakra (Anahata)

Located in the center of the chest, the heart chakra is ruled by air. It is associated with love, compassion, empathy, forgiveness, and relationships. When your heart chakra is blocked you feel jealous, closed off, antisocial, unforgiving, and overly defensive. You may feel a strong need for approval from others with a severe lack of self-esteem. You are unable to love yourself, so look to others to fulfill your need.

Cleanse your heart chakra by visualizing streaks of white light racing into your body through your outer appendages—your fingertips, your tippy toes, the crown chakra just at the top of your head. It penetrates your body, following ley lines to reach your heart chakra in the center of your chest. The white light flows into the chakra and begins spiraling, cleansing, rebalancing as it goes. The light changes into a bright green. The spiraling increases as energy radiates outward. The spiraling gently slows to a comfortable pulse, still shining bright. You are balanced and cleansed.

Throat Chakra (Vishuddha)

The throat chakra is located in the middle of your neck where your throat is. It is associated with your communication and expressive abilities. It is connected to creativity, same as the chakras below it and tied to spirit the same as the chakras above it. Imbalances or blockages in this chakra can cause you to talk too much or say the wrong thing. Your filter is shut off. Alternatively, you may be afraid to speak. Honesty and keeping your word become problematic.

Cleanse your throat chakra by visualizing streaks of white light racing into your body through your outer appendages—your fingertips, your tippy toes, the crown chakra just at the top of your head. It penetrates your body, following ley lines to reach your throat chakra in the center of your neck. The white light flows into the chakra and begins spiraling, cleansing, rebalancing as it goes. The light changes into a rich blue. The spiraling increases as energy radiates outward like waves. The spiraling gently slows to a comfortable pulse, still shining bright. You are balanced and cleansed.

Third Eye Chakra (Ajna)

The third eye chakra is located on the forehead in between your eyebrows. This is the home of your intuition, wisdom, and psychic abilities, which assist in your connection to spirit. A blockage or imbalance in the third eye chakra results in confusion, brain fog, and a disconnect with spirit. Your third eye chakra is a necessary part of your connections with deity, the universe, or oneness. An imbalance makes these connections impossible.

Cleanse your third eye chakra by visualizing streaks of white light racing into your body through your outer appendages—your fingertips, your tippy toes, the crown chakra just at the top of your head. It penetrates your body, following ley lines to reach your Ajna chakra in between your eyebrows, just above the bridge of your nose. The white light flows into the chakra and begins spiraling, cleansing, rebalancing as it goes. The light changes into a royal purple. The spiraling increases as energy radiates outward. The spiraling gently slows to a comfortable pulse, still shining bright. You are balanced and cleansed.

Crown Chakra (Sahasrara)

The crown chakra sits at the top of your head and radiates outward—like a crown. It is the center of your awareness, your higher consciousness. It is the blissful and sacred. While your third eye chakra helps guide you to spirit, it is in your crown chakra where oneness with the universe occurs. A blockage in either the third eye or crown chakras will impair your ability to hit a peak experience; an imbalance may cause a disconnect with your body. You become closed-minded and distant.

Cleanse your crown chakra by visualizing streaks of white light racing into your body through your outer appendages—your fingertips, your tippy toes. White light shoots down from above your crown chakra. It penetrates your body, following ley lines to reach your root chakra at the base of your spine. It spirals through the root chakra, then the sacral chakra, the solar plexus chakra, the heart chakra, the throat chakra, the third eye chakra, and up into the crown chakra. The spiraling increases as energy radiates outward—a bright white light encompassing all of you. The spiraling gently slows to a comfortable pulse, shrinking back down to the crown chakra, still shining bright. You are balanced and cleansed.

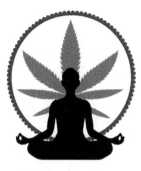

Conclusion

I completed the first round of edits on this book a matter of days before *Wake, Bake & Meditate: Take Your Spiritual Practice to a Higher Level with Cannabis* was released on May 8, 2020. As I sat and wrote this, the release was just over a week away. We had also been on lockdown for Covid 19 for seven weeks. By the time I began the final edits, it was July 2020 and over 140,000 Americans had lost their lives to this virus. It feels as if our country is being torn into two.

I tell you this as a reminder. Our world is forever changing. Our views change, society changes. What was normal when I began writing this book is nowhere near what we see as normal right now. By the time this book is published, I imagine we will be living in a completely new normal.

Because our world and our views change, you can use this book from year to year to year, repeating meditations whenever you like. Feelings, emotions, and thoughts prompted by a meditation in 2021 may be altogether different from performing the same meditation in 2029.

I pray the "new normal" our world finds is one that learns to value life over money and realizes people are our greatest treasure, resource, asset, and hope for a better future. I wish for a future filled with kindness, openness, and love. A future free of hate and despair.

A future I believe, and I hope you do too, cannabis needs to play a significant role in. Perhaps if more people used cannabis to heal their spiritual selves, healing society would be far more commonplace.

We must heal ourselves to be able to heal the world around us. We are one and the same.

I would like to thank you once again for joining me on this journey.

Go with peace, love, and happiness.

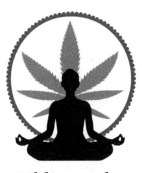

Bibliography

Barrons, Callie. "25 Inspirational Quotes About Weed."
    High Times. June 22, 2018. https://hightimes.com
    /culture/inspirational-quotes-about-weed/8/.

Black, Anna. *A Year of Living Mindfully: Week-by-Week
    Mindfulness Meditations for a More Contented and
    Fulfilled Life.* New York: Cico Books, 2015.

Blunts, Holden. *The Quotable Stoner: More Than 1,100
    Baked, Lit-Up, and Zonked-Out Quotes in Tribute
    to (And As a Result of) Smoking Weed.* Avon, MA:
    Adams Media, 2011.

Calaprice, Alice. *The Ultimate Quotable Einstein.* Princ-
    eton, NJ: Princeton University Press, 2011.

Caroline Caldwell. "In a society that profits from your self doubt, liking your self is a rebellious act." Twitter. May 17, 2015. https://twitter.com/dirt_worship/status /600028189113581569?lang=en.

Conway, D.J. *Moon Magick: Myth & Magick, Crafts & Recipes, Rituals & Spells*. St. Paul, MN: Llewellyn Publications, 1995.

Dyer, Wayne W. *Your Sacred Self: Making the Decision to Be Free*. New York: HarperCollins Publishers, 1995.

Ferrara, Mark S. "Peak Experiences and the Ineffable." In *Sacred Bliss: A Spiritual History of Cannabis*. 99–118. Rowman & Littlefield, 2018.

Gray, Stephen, ed. *Cannabis and Spirituality: An Explorer's Guide to an Ancient Plant Spirit Ally*. Rochester, VT: Park Street Press, 2017.

Grinspoon, Lester. *Marihuana Reconsidered*. Cambridge, MA: Harvard University Press, 1977.

Hanh, Thich Nhat. *The Art of Living: Peace and Freedom in the Here and Now*. New York: HarperOne, 2017.

Hoffman, Alice. *Practical Magic*. New York: Penguin, 2003.

"Hunter S Thompson: In His Own Words," *The Guardian*, February 21, 2005, https://www.theguardian.com /books/2005/feb/21/huntersthompson.

Lao Tzu, *The Tao Te Ching of Lao Tzu*. Translated by Brian Browne Walker. St. Martin's Press, 1995.

Lawrence, D. H. *The Collected Works of D. H. Lawrence.* Hastings, UK: Delphi Classics, 2015.

Marley, Bob, and Ian McCann. *Bob Marley "Talking": Bob Marley in His Own Words.* London: Omnibus Press, 2003.

Mehta, Viral. "Lessons in Living on the Edge From Mahatma Gandhi." Huffpost. August 31, 2011. https://www.huffpost.com/entry/selfless-action_b_940035.

Parker, Maggie. "13 of Audrey Hepburn's Most Inspiring Quotes." Time. May 4, 2016. https://time.com/4316700/audrey-hepburn-inspiring-quotes/.

Quindlen, Anna. *Being Perfect.* New York: Random House, 2005.

Simpson, Liz, and Patricia Mercier. *Chakra for Everyday Living.* Vacaville CA: Bounty Books, 2015.

Star Wars: Episode IV—A New Hope. Directed by George Lucas. 1977; Lucasfilm, Twentieth Century Fox.

Tolle, Eckhart. *The Power of Now: A Guide to Spiritual Enlightenment.* Hachette Australia, 2018.

"What Is a Black Moon?" *The Old Farmer's Almanac.* Yankee Publishing Inc. July, 31 2019. www.almanac.com/news/astronomy/astronomy/what-black-moon.

To Write to the Author

If you wish to contact the author or would like more information about this book, please write to the author in care of Llewellyn Worldwide Ltd. and we will forward your request. Both the author and publisher appreciate hearing from you and learning of your enjoyment of this book and how it has helped you. Llewellyn Worldwide Ltd. cannot guarantee that every letter written to the author can be answered, but all will be forwarded. Please write to:

Kerri Connor
℅ Llewellyn Worldwide
2143 Wooddale Drive
Woodbury, MN 55125-2989

Please enclose a self-addressed stamped envelope for reply, or $1.00 to cover costs. If outside the U.S.A., enclose an international postal reply coupon.

Many of Llewellyn's authors have websites with additional information and resources. For more information, please visit our website at http://www.llewellyn.com